T0209088

Praise for <u>Understanding Aging</u>

"Dr. Martin Terplan's pragmatic brilliance shines with this book about understanding aging. Compiled in four sections, this concise book artfully clarifies problems of aging and skillfully provides guidance. A great read."

Maryam Ziaie Matin, M.D.,F.A.C.P.
Internal Medicine and Geriatrics
San Francisco

"This is a great book. I wish I had it for my geriatric patients."

Richard M. Dennes, M.D.
Retired Nonagenarian
Internal Medicine and Geriatrics
Mill Valley, California

"Aging is something all of us encounter, if we are lucky. But no one wants to talk to us about what will happen, what to look out for, what to worry about, and what to ignore. It sneaks up on you. One day you notice a new pain, or some heavier breathing than you remember, or some dizziness. You could search magazines and the internet to find the cause, cure, and medication. You only have to decide which one actually applies.

This book cuts through all of this in an easy-to-read, well-organized way. It describes possible symptoms, what to expect, what to anticipate, what to seek help for.

It is not a self-help book, although it gives good hints on what you can do to improve. Its main purpose is to guide you through the possible changes in your aging body. It advises when you need medical attention or what alternatives you can explore in a light, understandable way. In addition to medical information, it provides good guidance on related issues like sleep, diet, health insurance, senior care facilities, money, and dying.

This insightful book should be required reading for everyone as they are getting old, or are planning to get old."

Peter K. Bohacek. Ph.D.
Octogenarian
New York City

"This was very enjoyable to read. I liked the straightforward advice and casual style. How less can be more in caring for the older adult makes this a practical guide on how to approach aging with dignity and grace."

Sarah Temkin, M.D., F.A.C.S.
Gynecologic Oncology
Washington, D.C.

"I was very impressed by <u>Understanding Aging</u>. It was very well-done, expressed in a style that is comprehensive, coherent, and understandable for all the aging people who need this useful information as life gets more and more complicated. It is enriched by the literary supplemental and poetic adages which grace each section. I actually learned a number of facts that I had ignored or missed on the way. (I'm aged 92.) If I had been so well-informed, I'm sure my present condition might well have been significantly benefited. But it's not too late.

I would urge all those who get to 60-70 to read this very cogent, helpful volume, which will enlighten and soften the oft-times rocky road and complex course of aging."

Jack Leibman, M.D.
Retired Internist
San Francisco

"Dr. Martin Terplan's book on aging is highly informative, concise, and clear. It is an excellent review of multiple medical and psychological aspects of aging, and is accessible to the average reader/patient as he/she deals with the multiple potential issues of aging. I highly recommend this book."

William J. Estrin, M.D.
Fellow of the American Academy of Neurology
San Francisco

UNDERSTANDING
AGING

A Resource for Living Better

Martin Terplan, M.D.

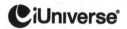

UNDERSTANDING AGING
A RESOURCE FOR LIVING BETTER

iUniverse books may be ordered through booksellers or by contacting:

iUniverse
1663 Liberty Drive
Bloomington, IN 47403
www.iuniverse.com
844-349-9409

ISBN: 978-1-6632-1366-2 (sc)
ISBN: 978-1-6632-1335-8 (e)

Library of Congress Control Number: 2020923133

Print information available on the last page.

iUniverse rev. date: 12/29/2020

CONTENTS

Preface ix

Section I   **WHAT CAUSES AGING?** 1

Chapter 1   Biological Influences 3
Chapter 2   Environmental and Social Influences 5

Section II   **WHAT ARE THE CLINICAL
            CONSEQUENCES OF AGING?** 7

Chapter 3   Extremities 9
    Bones 9
    Muscles 10
    Joints 10
    Hands and Wrists 12
    Elbows, Upper Arms, and Shoulders 13
    Hips 14
    Knees 14
    Ankles and Feet 15
    To Emphasize 16
Chapter 4   Spine 17
    Neck 18
    Thorax - The Upper Back 18
    Lumbar - The Lower Back 19
    Low Back Pain 20
    To Emphasize 21

Chapter 5   Organs of Sight, Hearing, Smell, and Taste 22
    Eyes - Common Disorders 22
    Ears - Hearing Impairment and Dizziness........................... 24
    Nose 25
    Mouth and Throat.. 26
    To Emphasize 27
Chapter 6   Lungs... 28
    Pneumonia... 29
    Emphysema and Other Chest Problems 30
    To Emphasize 31
Chapter 7   Heart and Blood Vessels 32
    Artery Disorders and Hypertension.................................. 32
    Vein Disorders 34
    Heart Valve Disorders 35
    Heart Rhythm Disorders 36
    Heart Attack and Heart Failure 37
    To Emphasize 38
Chapter 8   Gastrointestinal Tract 39
    Esophagus - Swallowing Problems 39
    Stomach and Small Intestines 41
    Colon and Rectum 42
    Liver and Gall Bladder... 43
    To Emphasize 43
Chapter 9   Genitourinary System in Men and Women........... 44
    Incontinence 44
    Prostate... 45
    Impotence or Erectile Dysfunction 46
    Gynecology.. 47
    To Emphasize 49
Chapter 10   Endocrine Disorders and Diabetes 50
    To Emphasize 51
Chapter 11   Brain and Nervous System.................................. 52
    Dementia - Memory Loss 52
    Alzheimer's Disease... 53
    Alzheimer Treatment 54

Parkinson's Disease 56
Stroke 57
Headache, Nerves, and Myalgia 58
To Emphasize 60
Chapter 12 Psychiatric Problems 61
To Emphasize 63
Chapter 13 Skin 64
Sun Damage and Tumors 65
Skin Infections 66
Scalp Hair Loss 67
To Emphasize 67

Section III **WHAT EXTERNAL INFLUENCES
AFFECT THE ELDERLY?** 69

Chapter 14 Health Care 71
Office Visit 71
Routine Health-Care Expenses 73
Hospital-Level Care 73
Post-Hospital Care 76
To Emphasize 77
Chapter 15 Cancer 78
To Emphasize 80
Chapter 16 Infections 81
To Emphasize 83
Chapter 17 Pills 84
Prescription Drugs 84
Non-Prescription Drugs 85
Use and Misuse of Pills 85
Drug Companies 86
To Emphasize 87
Chapter 18 Diet 88
Fruits and Vegetables 88
Meat and Fish 90
To Emphasize 91

Chapter 19   Addictions 92
    Alcohol 92
    Drugs.. 93
    To Emphasize 94
Chapter 20   Sleep - Wakefulness and Dreams 95
    Sleeping Pills... 95
    Sleep Problems.. 96
    To Emphasize 97
Chapter 21   Exercise.. 98
    Muscle Exercises 98
    Balance Exercises 100
    To Emphasize 101
Chapter 22   Money 102
    Use and Misuse 102
    Money in Insurance.. 102
    Money in Health Care 103
    Money in Pharma 105
    Money in Employment 105
    To Emphasize 106

Section IV   **WHAT HAPPENS TOWARDS THE
                 END OF LIFE?**.. 107

Chapter 23   Home Care or Assisted Living 109
    Living at Home... 109
    Home Help... 110
    Assisted Living.. 111
Chapter 24   Nursing Homes 113
    Nursing Home Care 114
    COVID-19 and Nursing Homes...115
    Unresponsive Patients 116
Chapter 25   Death and Dying.. 118
    Trying to Understand Death.. 119
    Certifying Death 121

Closing Thoughts.. 125
Acknowledgements.. 133

PREFACE

Why this book? Why now?

In most westernized countries, the birthrate has fallen, while increasing numbers of their citizens enter a geriatric age group. In the United States during each recent decade, the percentage of older people has grown.

When I retired from my private medical practice in 2013, and from teaching at the University of California in San Francisco, I became one of those older people I was going to write about. I found myself in a position common to many older Americans. I needed to find a primary care doctor, and I needed to find affordable healthcare insurance. Medicare had protected me from high hospital expenses, and medical colleagues had been available for specific needs. No longer. Private care doctors had either joined groups or restricted themselves to a "boutique" practice, one in which a physician would provide all care for a fixed fee. Medicare alone was not enough to enable me to enroll in these practices. I had to choose among a somewhat bewildering array of medical plans. Making choices is part of life, and, as I noticed, at least in healthcare, costs more.

My new doctor, a skilled internist, commented one day about how her practice had begun to contain ever more older patients. She had increasingly become a geriatrician, but on looking for pamphlets or publications which would enable her patients to understand their aging, to help them cope better, she found none. She implied that, with my background, I might help her supply one.

I went into local bookstores and found that she was right. There were plenty of books about how to live longer, about lifestyle modifications, spiritual growth, exercise programs, dietary changes, but no comprehensive book enabling patients to understand their own healthcare problems, the ones aging created.

So the answer to why this book, and why now, is to fill a need for this expanding group of older people.

Looking further, I found there were always books of varying quality concerning the elderly. As early as the 16th century, one could read about old people, about their healthcare problems, and one could even have read a critique of geriatric literature available at that time.

As quoted by John H. Talbott, M.D., in A Biographical History of Medicine (Grune & Stratton, Inc.:1970), Francois Rauchin, who was born in Montpelier, France, in 1560, wrote:

"Not only physicians, but everybody else attending old people, being accustomed to their constant complaints and knowing their ill-tempered and difficult manners, realized how noble and important, how serious and difficult, how useful, and even indispensable is that part of practical medicine called geriatrics, which deals with the conservation of old people and the healing of their diseases.

Its indispensability results from the deficiencies of nature, because of the hardships, the pains, the weaknesses, with which old people are afflicted, almost without interruptions.

Its usefulness is demonstrated by consideration of the political fact that the administration of economical matters depends on the conservation of old people."

So Rauchin wrote that 400 years ago, in France, his patients were complainers, ill-tempered, difficult, peevish; they were afflicted by almost uninterrupted pains and weaknesses. Today's patients have the same ills, but, in my practice at least, I rarely saw patients I could have described as ill-tempered, difficult, or peevish. Life has changed profoundly in the past 400 years. The manner of speaking has changed, as well. Complainers exist but are not so widespread, except perhaps among some of the very old.

Rauchin also noted the political fact that, administratively, the economy had to take into account the conservation of old people. Our governments must do the same, indeed increasingly so, as more and more older people survive. What will we do now with burgeoning numbers of old people? Will they be an asset or a liability? It is clear that they need more attention, more services as they age. Can we provide them? One measure of a society or of a country is how it takes care of its most vulnerable. How will we fare?

Japan, a nation with an already high percentage of an older population, hosted a Super Aging international conference in October, 2019, so aware were they of the need to prepare intelligently for the impact that increasing numbers of very old individuals would have. Even though they noted that 90% of employees of a large company retired when eligible to do so at age 65, the government was still striving to create a society of free choice, a society that enabled people to work their entire lives, if they so wished. They were catering to the observation that because some workers feel adrift when no longer gainfully employed, no longer contributing to society, many chose to continue working.

Finally, Rauchin went on to comment that the difficulty of aging, "is shown, not only by the peevishness of old people, but especially by the fact that this science has been neglected by our forefathers, and even by modern authors, too. What has been written about the conservation of old people and the healing of diseases of old age is so bad and so unproductive that we get the impression that it has been flatly suppressed and buried."

His observations concerning his contemporary physician authors is striking, and even amusing. Authors must have been different 400 years ago, but our modern authors today do not suppress or bury issues related to geriatric health. When they write, they write about and describe the same ills that existed not only 400 years ago but 800 and 1,600 years ago as well. Circumstances change, but as Mark Twain observed, human nature doesn't. Older patients now arise in vastly different surroundings, but their symptoms remain the same.

Aging changes everything, but, at least at first, slowly. We see it in ourselves, and I saw it in patients. Once healthy middle-aged men and women would gradually appear with a new concern, a problem that might not disappear—a symptom, a discomfort, an illness, one that seemed to belong almost exclusively to an older age group. (My younger patients usually had different complaints.) The new complaints of these older patients began to define the kind of limitations they might have, indeed limitations that an older person, sooner or later, could expect to have. One example, out of many, is their vulnerability to infections. These infections arise more readily and heal more slowly. They are also more lethal. Witness COVID-19.

The challenge this book proposes is to clarify what symptoms, what problems arise with aging, while providing advice and a resource for both patients and their caregivers, with the overall goal of helping the patient understand his or her own aging and thereby live more wisely.

Bob Feller, a top pitcher for the Cleveland Indians baseball team in the mid-20th century, announced one day that he had leukemia. He was in his early 90s, but he said that he would "still like to live a little longer on this side of the grass." It is a great expression, most of us at the end of our lives might agree, but not all. We will see why.

This book is divided into the following topics:

SECTION I: WHAT CAUSES AGING?

SECTION II. WHAT ARE THE CLINICAL CONSEQUENCES OF AGING?

SECTION III. WHAT EXTERNAL INFLUENCES AFFECT AGING?

SECTION IV: WHAT HAPPENS TOWARDS THE END OF LIFE?

CLOSING THOUGHTS

SECTION I

WHAT CAUSES AGING?

Millennia of adaptations have made man essentially stable and healthy. When intrusions such as cuts, bruises, infections, stomach upsets, indeed any kind of perturbation occurred, body defense mechanisms were enlisted to try and restore normalcy. Do nothing, use common sense, and you would usually get better. "God heals," they said, "and the doctor takes the fee."

Despite accumulated birthdays, wrinkles, scalp hair changes, a slower climb up stairs, you remained basically fit. If you thought about getting old at all, and now and then you certainly did, you felt yourself fortunate. And one day, you were surprised when somebody offered you a seat on the bus, which you politely refused. That was Stage One of aging. In Stage Two, you took the seat. You accepted what everyone else had already recognized: Your body had aged. You were old. The determinants of this aging were the cumulative effects of biological, environmental, and social disruptions on your body. They affect everyone.

CHAPTER 1

BIOLOGICAL INFLUENCES

Theories exist to explain the biological changes resulting in aging. We understand many of these changes but not yet all of them. (Some changes are known, but no proven mechanisms exist.) After our bodies are fully grown, cellular activity still continues, essentially unchanged. There is just no new net growth of the total number of cells. With aging, some cells die and are not replaced. And there is an increased propensity to accumulate senescent cells, older ones, perhaps slightly defective ones.

Cells are the fundamental structure in our body, each with a cell membrane and a nucleus containing genetic material and DNA. Throughout life, cells renew themselves, removing the old by splitting and regenerating a new cell, the exact copy of the old. The energy for this metabolic activity derives from oxygen, water, and food, with these nutrients delivered to the cells by blood circulation. It goes on continuously.

Is there a limit to this process of cell division and regeneration? The answer is yes; the number of times a human fibroblast reproduced itself was once measured at 72 times. There are surely differences in other cells, and among different individuals, but our body cannot indefinitely replace cells with viable new ones. Before that process stops, however, you will already have died.

With time, cell reproduction falters, cells are not always replaced,

3

and little by little shrinking occurs. In old age, there are fewer kidney cells, fewer muscle cells, fewer neurons. With fewer cells, our organs shrink. We tend to lose weight. We lose muscle and bone, but proportionately less fat, hence the percentage of body fat rises, and, if there is any fat visible, it is, of course, at the waistline. We look smaller, and we are.

Moreover, continual cell splitting will ultimately result in some errors, sometimes repairable, sometimes not. Affected cells function less efficiently. Chromosomal abnormalities which arise can be minor, or they can be major and initiate a whole new cell line growth, benign perhaps, or malignant, with the resultant cancer, sometimes easy to treat, often not.

While all this cellular activity is going on, our organs are also getting older. Hearts pump less efficiently, lung capacity lessens, our kidneys and livers eliminate body toxins less well, and our brains send and receive messages more slowly. Arterial depositions of cholesterol and calcium increase. Our arteries have hardened. Every part of our body functions less well. We are less resilient.

Our aging cells have begun to receive decreasing nourishment. We have become vulnerable to superimposed fatal events. We don't die from old age alone, but rather from an accident, or a disease, cancer, an infection, or a cardiovascular event. Whatever it is, we can no longer overcome it.

CHAPTER 2

ENVIRONMENTAL AND SOCIAL INFLUENCES

While it is very unlikely that biological changes underlying aging have changed in millennia, and very likely that a similar proportion of individuals in every society reach a very old age, a healthy environment was always the major determinant of longevity. Indeed, if men could have avoided wars and women could have avoided obstetrical problems, everyone with access to healthy water had an equal opportunity for a long life.

But the environment always interfered. Water pollution did occur, industrial smog befouled the air, contaminants, even carcinogens, entered the food chain. While man was overcoming one problem, others kept arising. An epidemic happened, or a war occurred. Yet in many countries, man kept ahead. During the last century, life expectancy has increased in many societies, the major reason being better public health. As the environment became healthier, people became healthier and lived longer.

One other environmental factor affecting aging is the early health of each person. Good health is not uniformly distributed. Some suffer minor or major problems early in life, which become chronic impediments. Each one so burdened must learn to live with the consequences. They don't necessarily impact longevity, but when they do, they bring about aging earlier than otherwise.

We want to believe that every baby born, every human being, has an equal chance in life, equal opportunities in the pursuit of self-fulfillment and happiness, but they don't.

Whether we like it or not, individuals belonging to a higher socioeconomic class tend to live longer and healthier. Why? It is not because they do less physical work, for physical activity in a healthy environment should be good, but rather because they have more choices about their lives.

They can avoid living next to an oil refinery. They can choose a neighborhood with good schools. They have better access to healthcare. They are better educated. They are better informed; thus they tend to avoid smoking, drugs, and alcohol abuse. Their neighborhoods have fewer gun wars, less crime, fewer accidents. They are more removed from poverty, from homelessness. In short, their very real social advantages protect them from some of the adverse effects society would otherwise impose on their aging process.

Due to socioeconomic differences, geographic variations in morbidity and mortality exist everywhere. In Norway, for example, the life expectancy of the poorest 1% of men in 2015 was 13.8 years shorter than the wealthiest 1%. The comparable difference for women was 8.4 years (Journal of the American Medical Association, May 21, 2019).

Alcoholism, substance abuse, smoking, poverty, educational deprivation, singly or in combination, underlie the social dislocation which many individuals suffer, and they impact aging. They shorten lives. And, unfortunately, they are difficult to control.

SECTION II

WHAT ARE THE CLINICAL CONSEQUENCES OF AGING?

The following eleven chapters describe the influence of aging on the structure and function of each body part. They present the symptoms which arise and their subsequent management. Everyone will have many of these changes. No one will have all.

CHAPTER 3

EXTREMITIES

ANATOMICAL CHANGES, FRACTURES, ARTHRITIS

Your extremities are your organs of locomotion. They consist of bones, muscles, ligaments, joints, nerves. They move things around. Their conductor is in your brain.

Bones

Just like cellular activity in the rest of the body, your bone cells constantly renew themselves, osteoclasts breaking down and eliminating bone, osteoblasts rebuilding bone. Exercise, hormones, calcium, and vitamin D all influence this process. Even gravitational force affects bone metabolism. At zero gravity, for example, astronauts with no force on their bones while in space uniformly lose bone.

With aging, this continual bone modeling favors bone loss. Your arms and legs do not get shorter (height loss with age is due to spine shortening), but they get weaker. X-rays will show a loss of bone tissue, as will bone density studies. Bone loss occurs proportionately each year. Hence, if you begin adulthood heavier with thicker bones, it will take longer for your bones to become significantly osteoporotic. But if you are slightly built, be careful. Your bones will break more readily.

Muscles

Meanwhile, your muscles have been losing mass by failing to renew lost muscle fibers. You have become weaker, each decade more so. The weights you can carry or the stairs you can climb are fewer. Trying to slow down this muscle loss with exercise is always a good idea and helps, but you cannot regain the bulk you once had. Similarly, the tissues and fibers under your skin have been disappearing, resulting in thinner skin. Just compare your hands and forearms to those of a young adult, and you will see how visible your tendons and blood vessels have become. And compare your upper arms and shoulders with your younger self to notice how more prominent your bones look, how much muscle you have lost.

The net result of tissue, muscle, and bone loss is increased weakness with a corresponding increased chance of injury. Whereas a young person can fall without injury, even minor falls can cause major fractures or disability in the elderly. Therefore, and you will hear this again: TAKE CARE. HOLD ON. DON'T FALL.

Joints

The components that make up your joints also age. Typically, a joint connects two bones held together by surrounding ligaments and tendons, and in the hips and shoulders, by muscles as well. Cartilage lines the bony surface of the joint, and a thin synovial membrane, which secretes nutrients into the joint space, surrounds the joint.

Joints, moving over many decades, wear down, lose fibers, develop tears. They become slightly tighter and distorted. Calcium depositions might appear, compensatory bony growth arises, and the disfigured appearance is called arthritis, more accurately, degenerative arthritis or osteoarthritis. In spite of the suffix "-itis," which indicates inflammation, there is no inflammatory disease. Joint mobility is reduced, but at rest there is little or no pain.

There are other forms of arthritis that are not specifically related to aging, even though they may become more prevalent with age. These are most notably rheumatoid due to auto-immune factors, gouty or gout-like due to metabolic abnormalities, and infectious arthritis due to bacterial contamination. They all require medical consultation for diagnosis and therapy.

Your extremities are also prone to sprains and strains. What is the difference? A sprain involves an injury to ligaments surrounding a joint. A forceful stretching causes tears, broken capillaries, and a body reaction resulting in fluid accumulating within the joint space and surrounding area, producing swelling and pain.

Strains, on the other hand, involve muscles or tendons. Overuse of a muscle group would tend to fatigue and shorten its muscle bundles, placing more tension on their tendons, thereby straining the area. Muscle strains also arise from an unexpected pull on a muscle group, causing some muscle fibers to tear.

To maintain bone health, muscle health, tissue health, joint health, and to keep strong, stretch and exercise regularly. Placing a force on bones retards bone loss. Just walking for your legs and carrying groceries for your arms may be enough. Adequate dietary calcium and vitamin D (1,200 mg of calcium, 800 International Units (IU) of Vitamin D daily), which most normal diets provide, are also required for healthy bones. Medications are usually not necessary.

And remember to treat problems promptly. Delaying simply prolongs recovery. You can treat most sprains and strains yourself, ideally by icing and compressing the involved area immediately after the injury, in order to reduce swelling, and then gradually stretching the area more and more over ensuing days. Heat or a Jacuzzi might help with comfort and healing.

Most fractures, major joint injuries, and persistent unexplained joint swelling or tenderness will need medical attention for diagnosis and treatment. If an initial x-ray discloses no problem, but one point over the site remains tender to pressure, a later x-ray or other study will often show a hairline fracture needing care.

Hands and Wrists

Look at your hands, and if you are old enough, you will see arthritis. It may be as little as small bony nodules at the side of your last joint (the distal interphalangeal) in the second, third, fourth or fifth finger. These deformities are called Heberden's nodes and are essentially asymptomatic. The next joint (the proximal interphalangeal) may also be involved and distorted. Indeed, both joints could become very distorted with loss of mobility but with usually no more than mild discomfort on use, or mild disability on use. The only other common joint involved by the same arthritic process is in the joint connecting the base of your thumb to your wrist. If it is involved, you will note a slight protuberance there, and some minor discomfort on pressure. Neither medications, ointments, or physiotherapy will retard the osteoarthritic process, nor will they help your minor symptoms. You can try stretching the involved joints on a daily basis, which should improve mobility and might slow down the developing deformity.

The elderly are particularly prone to a sympathetic nerve dysfunction, more recently named complex regional pain syndrome (CRPS), primarily involving the hand following upper arm injuries or fractures. The fingers may become stiffer with some loss of flexion, and the hand can be painful, moist, and cool. There are physical therapists and occupational therapists who specialize in trying to restore normal hand function. CRPS is exceedingly difficult to cure, but therapists definitely help ameliorate the symptoms and make the syndrome generally manageable for most patients.

Wrists have far fewer arthritic problems, but they are perhaps more exposed to trauma. If you fall, your immediate reflex reaction is to soften the blow with outstretched hands, thus creating an upward force on your wrist and arm. If the force at your wrist is strong enough, and the bone of your distal radius weak enough, the bone will break (termed a Colles fracture). You will need medical attention.

Lesser impacts such as over-stretching at the wrist can result in a sprained wrist. Repeated twisting motions can strain ligaments. Direct blows can cause soft tissue injuries. With rest, you can usually manage all these at home.

Elbows, Upper Arms, and Shoulders

Tennis elbows and similar repetitive swinging actions at the elbow can strain aging muscles or tendons, producing discomfort where the tendons attach at either side of the elbow. Stopping or changing the provoking activity helps. It will soon go away, but, if not, it might require a cortisone injection.

The tip of the elbow (the olecranon process) contains a small protective lubricating lining called a bursa. Repeated pressure over this area can produce irritation with fluid filling this space, resulting in a bursitis. Rest relieves, but occasionally medical attention is required to drain the fluid.

Falls directly onto the elbow can also break bones. The older you are, the more difficult it will be to avoid some disability after treatment. Be prepared.

The upper arm (the humerus) and the clavicle both form part of the shoulder joint and can fracture from falls. The rotator cuff (a group of tendons in front of and above the joint) is responsible for all the rotation motion at the shoulder, and with injury it can become frayed or develop tears. Even without an obvious injury, you may begin to notice difficulty raising your arm above your head, or performing similar rotations. Stretching and perhaps physical therapy (PT) will always help. Even if a tendon is completely severed,

13

PT alone can often restore up to 95% of former use. You may not need surgery.

Avoid one other common problem—a frozen shoulder. Not using the shoulder due to injuries or illness can result in tendon tightness, impairing subsequent shoulder rotation, sometimes impairing it very greatly. By simply rotating your upper arms every day with motions simulating swimming, you should be able to avoid problems.

Hips

The hip is so well protected by encasing muscles that it takes quite a blow to create injury. But once again, aging makes the hip vulnerable to fracture by these two common perils: osteoporosis and falls. Women, with their greater tendency to have osteoporosis, are particularly vulnerable. The incidence of osteoporotic hip fracture increases with age to the extent that the thinner neck of the femur (thigh bone) can fracture with a very minimal fall. Hip fractures are common, and, in very old patients, may prevent walking thereafter despite excellent treatment. Know, though, that hip replacement surgery, or most elective surgeries for hip problems, are successful, and after a period of recovery, most patients will walk well, though it may take weeks to months.

Knees

Increased cartilage loss within the knee joint and pathologic processes that involve subchondral bone, synovium, and menisci accompany aging. The joint space becomes narrowed, enabling the bone from the thigh to rub on the lower leg bone. Hence, if you get old enough, you probably will have discomfort, more walking downhill than uphill. Why? Because when you walk downhill, there is more force on your knee joint, the force of gravity being added to the full weight of your body - one reason why these cartilage changes develop in the first place. Thus, the heavier you are, the more you have pounded your knee over a lifetime, the more likely you will suffer cartilage loss, ultimately to the extent that the resultant bony irritation will limit your walking.

There will alway be a few individuals whose knees don't bother them much, who play tennis into their nineties. However, for most it is the major joint limiting activity, and its management involves exercise. The extensor muscles of your thigh (the quadriceps) are the largest in your body, and the stronger they are, the better they will stabilize your knee. Daily or near daily quadriceps exercises are essential, done most easily while lying down at home, and simply raising your legs multiple times, or done from a sitting position by extending your lower legs against gravity or against light weights. A simple way to construct a weight at home is to put a 2-3 pound rock at each end of a knee-length cotton sock and tie together the open end. Then simply place the "rock-sock" over your foot and raise it. From either a sitting or a lying position, you should also exercise the vastus medialis (a small muscle on the inner side of your knee). Tighten this muscle by hyperextending your knee. You will see your knee cap pulled upwards.

You should also use poles while hiking or walking on hills. In fact, you have probably seen some people already using them on city streets, as well. Proper use of poles will reduce the force on each knee with each step.

If all else fails, knee surgery is an option, as some of your acquaintances have surely already experienced.

Ankles and Feet

Ankle sprains and fractures can occur in any age group, and the treatments are the same for all. If you were able to strengthen the ligaments around your ankle by skating as a youngster, you will be better off now, but it is still not too late to incorporate ankle stretching to your daily exercise routine. Simply stand on your toes and rock back and forth onto your heels multiple times. Supportive shoes will also help prevent problems, particularly if you have ankle arthritis.

If you have worn tight shoes too long, you will see that your toes have crunched together, exposing the joint at the base of your great toe to more pressure. Your body responds by forming a callus (thickened skin). If the pressure is deeper and continues, bursitis forms, which can harden, resulting in a bunion. Nonetheless, avoid surgery; healing in the feet is poor. Special shoes help, and if you have good sensation in your feet, go barefoot more often.

With aging, there is also a loss of your heel pad or cushion because the heel ligaments containing the enclosed fat have stretched. When stepping down on a hard object, you are therefore apt to have pain. If this becomes a problem, plastic heel cups inserted into your shoes will help.

Finally, make sure you have normal feeling in your feet. Check your soles, for a common problem is to have reduced sensation and not notice that a small stone in your shoe, for example, has created a small ulcer. These ulcers become readily infected and take weeks of treatment to get better. As you know, prevention is better than cure.

Prevention is always better. The same applies to ingrown toenails or any visible irritation on your feet. Prevent minor common cuts or bruises or pressure points from getting worse. Inevitably, old feet have old circulation, and poor healing is the rule.

To Emphasize

1. Stretch joints daily.
2. Exercise muscles, particularly around creaky knees and sore shoulders.
3. Use hiking poles.

CHAPTER 4

SPINE
ANATOMY, FUNCTION, AND AGING DISORDERS

The spine extends from the skull to the sacrum and consists of a vertebral column, eight cervical, twelve thoracic, and five lumbar vertebrae. Because man is an upright animal, evolutionary adjustments led to the heaviest vertebrae becoming the lowest lumbar ones. This area, the third, fourth and fifth lumbar, continues to receive the most force over a lifetime in supporting an upright body, and it is here where most back problems arise.

The vertebral column contains the spinal cord, which ends at the first lumbar area, from where lower nerve roots descend. Nerve roots leave the vertebral column through an opening in each vertebral body, called a foramen, where problems often arise with aging. Arthritic changes reduce the foramen, thus more readily pinching the exiting nerve, often from a ruptured disc encroaching upon the site.

What is a ruptured disc? In the front of the spine, there is a disc-like shape between each bony vertebral body. The disc contains fluid in its interior which serves to cushion pressures on the spine. In time, fluid is lost, the disc becomes less resilient, and its fibrous surface more prone to defects. The disc material can then extrude through any defect; hence, the disc is ruptured, which, if pressing on a nerve root, causes pain. You often hear of people with "a slipped disc" or of their "back going out," but these are always inexact diagnoses.

Neck

Most neck problems are not due to the spine at all. They are muscle strains, shortening of muscle bundles, or spasms caused by remaining in a cramped position too long, for example, while sleeping. They can also arise from blows or from a sudden unexpected twisting motion at the neck. With appropriate exercise, stretching, perhaps heat, you should get better in time, but it may take two to three weeks. A not uncommon cause is sitting or sleeping with too many pillows under your head, creating excessive stretch on the muscles at the back of your neck. Use no more than one pillow. To try and prevent neck problems from arising in the first place, stretch your head in all directions as part of your daily exercise program. You can also try something more difficult: While lying on your back, try to support the full weight of your body with your head and feet only, lifting your torso off the floor. It is not easy, but the effort alone might help.

With persisting pain, particularly with radiation into your arms or with a loss of sensation, get professional help. Though not common, compression of a nerve root can occur in the neck (cervical) spine just as it does in the lumbar spine.

Thorax - The Upper Back

With age, everyone loses height due to compression, mainly of thoracic vertebral bodies or discs. Although an acute compression fracture of a vertebral body will cause pain, even severe pain, most compressions occur slowly and are asymptomatic. Often the major compression is in the front part of the vertebral body, causing the back to bend forward, most prominently in the upper back. Sometimes this spine curvature is marked enough to cause the cervical spine to compensate by extending the neck, thereby lifting the head in order to maintain forward vision. There is no corrective treatment, which is why you see so many older people with a rounded upper back. This slightly altered posture has the additional effect of shifting the body's center of gravity forward, causing sometimes mild muscle strains and a reduced sense of balance. If troubled with this postural change, putting on a backpack containing a few books will help.

I recall one woman in her late 80s, quite stooped, but quite energetic, who had consulted neck and shoulder specialists because of chronic discomforts. These symptoms remained unresolved until she added some bulk to the backpack she wore on her daily hikes. Doing so stretched her shoulders backwards, thus improving her center of gravity. With the added weight in her pack, moreover, her center of gravity moved even further backwards, and her balance improved as did her muscle strains. Backpack therapy works.

Lumbar - The Lower Back

In the lumbar spine, the effects of aging on the spine are most pronounced. Everyone has had an occasional low back spasm or pain. Everyone old enough has some limitations of movement. Everyone has some visible or x-ray evidence of deformity. What has happened? In addition to disc rupture, arthritic changes take place around the foramina or around any of the several joints connecting the vertebrae to one another. As these changes are not equal bilaterally, there is usually one side of the spine more bent than the other. When you look at yourself in a mirror, your lower back might look quite distorted, one hip higher than the other, or there might be a serious inability to stand straight. Muscles, ligaments, and tendons become differently stressed, and discomfort ensues. Nevertheless, you will usually improve with exercise, posture control, and time. Sometimes, though, the arthritic changes begin to compress the spinal cord or nerves, in which case surgery may help. The verb is "may help." In general, try to avoid spine surgery unless nerve loss is imminent.

You can do some tests yourself. If straight leg raising, one side or the other, causes back pain, you may be stretching a spinal nerve against the foramen opening. Irritation of the nerve causes an inflammatory body response as a reaction to the irritation. This is a useful response, but it comes with swelling, which may temporarily increase pressure at the site, causing more discomfort. You will need to rest the area for a short while.

Low Back Pain

The best thing to do for lower back pain is exercise and patience. In time you will improve. Both for prevention and treatment, specific back exercises are useful, and posture control is essential. Try this: While standing, stretch your back in all directions. Then kneel on the floor with your toes stretched out and your buttocks over your heels. Bring your chest down to the floor. You will feel stretching in your lower back. Hold this position for one minute or so. Then lie flat on your abdomen and try to raise your chest and your legs from the floor simultaneously, thus supporting yourself on your abdomen alone. It is not easy, but just trying will help.

Thereafter, roll onto your back, and do pelvic tilts by sucking your stomach in while thrusting your pelvis forward. You can also do these pelvic tilt exercises during the day while sitting or standing. Finish the back floor exercises with sit-ups, for strong abdominal muscles will support your back.

One day, I advised this exercise program to a woman who told me her husband was confined at home with a recurrent back problem. When she heard that part of the treatment required his being on the floor, she laughed and said, "If he got down to the floor, he might never get up."

This brings up another problem. Be certain you can always get back on your feet should you ever trip and fall, or somehow end up on the floor or ground. Whatever movement you may have to do, which might include crawling until you find a bench, make sure you do something in order to be able to rise onto your feet again. You don't want to be left alone for prolonged periods of time on the ground or on the floor.

To Emphasize

1. Stand straight. Sit straight. Don't slouch.
2. Stretch your lower back daily.
3. Do sit-ups.

CHAPTER 5

ORGANS OF SIGHT, HEARING, SMELL, AND TASTE

Man ascended from the sea. When we now enter the sea, it bathes our body, our eyes, our nose and mouth. It does no harm. It might even be helpful. I often wondered if its salt content impeded the growth of harmful bacteria or viruses. In fact, I usually advised patients to gargle with warmed salt water for sore throats or sniff warmed salt water for colds or sinus infections. Moreover, human tears are a weak salt solution, seemingly anti-septic for eyes.

Lately, I've begun to wonder if individuals exposed to sea water have a lower incidence of COVID-19 infection. It's pure speculation. An environmental study to test any such hypothesis would be impossible to conduct, as many, if not most, patients with COVID-19 had conditions making ocean beach use unlikely.

Do the viruses causing COVID-19 or influenzas grow in seawater? I can't find the answer. Meanwhile, if done easily enough, a salt water rinse of mouth and throat after exposure to someone with a viral upper respiratory infection is unlikely to harm.

Eyes - Common Disorders

The tiny muscles controlling the shape of your lens in each eye become weaker with age, just like every other muscle in your body.

Ultimately, your ability to focus on near objects will change, and if you've never worn glasses before, you will soon have to purchase some. Paradoxically, if you were nearsighted before and required glasses, you may now note you can read without them. These visual changes you can handle yourself, but almost all others will need professional help.

Glaucoma is more common in aging, and often family-related. It is a slowly progressive, persisting elevation of intra-ocular pressure, affecting peripheral vision at first. Untreated, it will cause blindness. Ocular exams every one to five years, the exact interval dependent upon prior exams, will detect the problem and enable therapy.

In the elderly, degeneration of the macula, the central part of the retina, the area required for visual acuity, is the leading cause of visual loss in the United States. By age 75, almost 30% of individuals are affected. It is slowly progressive, a progress that ophthalmologists can sometimes slow down. Although treatment might help, there is nothing you can specifically do to prevent degeneration of the macula from arising.

A cataract is a lens opacity, usually bilateral. It is the leading cause of blindness worldwide because access to treatment is still limited in some areas of the globe. Cataract development due to aging is common; indeed, most people over age 65 have some degree of lens opacity. When it becomes severe enough, surgical replacement has become a frequent useful procedure.

Even though there is a genetic predisposition to cataracts, avoiding exposure to strong lights and wearing protective sunglasses will retard its development.

But just because you have a cataract does not mean you need surgery. Cataracts can be small, grow slowly, and barely interfere with vision or reading for long periods of time. Moreover, particularly for many older patients in whom surgery would help, practical impediments exist. For example, during surgery, patients must lie down flat and must try to keep their eyes and head still. After surgery, they will need eye drops, often several times a day. These problems are not insurmountable, but they must be considered if one decides to have cataract surgery.

Ears - Hearing Impairment and Dizziness

Hearing loss occurs progressively with aging, ultimately affecting up to half the population. No wonder there are so many advertisements for hearing aids. The usual cause is genetic predisposition, often combined with prolonged noise exposure.

The energy of noise is measured in decibels. The decibel level of normal conversation is about 60, and levels exceeding 85 are injurious. When repeated often enough and long enough, auditory receptors become permanently damaged, initially interfering with hearing high frequency sound waves. Thereafter, there is gradual progression to lower frequency loss. Loss of speech discrimination, at least initially, is especially pronounced in noisy environments, before becoming noticeable in normal group conversations, and ultimately in face-to-face settings.

As soon as you notice some hearing loss, get professional help. Do not be vain about wearing a hearing aid. It helps. Moreover, the sooner you use one, the better you will hear, for if your brain begins missing sounds, it may not be able to recover those sounds later, even with hearing aids.

There are other causes of hearing loss from unusual disorders to simply impacted wax. For these, you will need help.

If impacted wax is a recurrent problem, and in some patients it frequently is, you or your caregiver can learn how to irrigate your ear canal. Unless you can see what you are doing, do not use cotton tips, for they will often push wax deeper into the canal.

Vertigo, a sensation of motion when there is no motion, is usually an ear problem, and dizziness is its major symptom. If you develop it, pay close attention to the symptoms, for light-headedness due to transient brain blood reduction can produce similar sensations.

Dizziness occurs when the fluid within the semicircular canals is set into motion. Should this occur by a tiny calcific piece breaking away from the side of the canal, the resulting diagnosis is called benign paroxysmal positioning vertigo. If dizziness persists or is recurrent enough, therapists can show you how to perform Epley exercises, transiently changing your head position to change the position of the offending calcified piece.

There are other causes of vertigo, including head trauma, labyrinthitis, and Ménière syndrome, all requiring professional help.

Nose

The paranasal sinuses, which drain into your nose, frequently become chronically congested, increasing secretions into your nose, which are then swept backwards into your throat. This so-called postnasal drip tends to puddle in the throat, provoking a cough. Common colds act similarly, and both are best treated with steam inhalations and sniffing. Blowing your nose, particularly hard blowing, increases the likelihood that some secretions get forced back into your sinuses or into your ear. You do not want this to happen because it can cause bacterial infections.

Follow any blowing by sniffing, which helps draw secretions out of your sinuses or your eustachian tubes. If your sinuses or nose still feel congested, sniff steam or draw warmed salt water into your nostrils

Should you ever have a nosebleed, simply press your nostrils together for five minutes. Most nosebleeds arise from the front of the nose, and after compression, the bleeding ordinarily stops without difficulty.

A problem peculiar to the elderly is a runny nose of clear watery secretions due to an increased sensitivity of nerves within the nose to such stimuli as air temperature change or scents. It can provoke loud sneezes, as well. The diagnosis is vasomotor rhinitis; it is not to be confused with allergic rhinitis or hay fever, and it requires no treatment. Indeed, it has no treatment.

Aging also reduces your sense of smell. The olfactory receptors in your nose no longer function as efficiently as they once did. Test this by trying to sniff a rose.

Mouth and Throat

You also have many fewer taste buds, and, since taste also involves smell, it is claimed that your ability to taste foods is no longer as acute. This is a difficult proposition to test, but when accompanied by your reduced sense of smell, you may well be able to enjoy a cheaper bottle of wine just as much as a more expensive one. Growing older does have some financial advantages.

Mouth secretions diminish with age. A dry mouth becomes more common, and gum infections more likely. Make sure to drink enough water, and continue dental hygiene. Your teeth also will have a tendency to migrate towards the midline, exposing more gum surfaces, and the pockets you have had may become deeper. Avoid tooth loss, yet some root infections may best be treated by extraction without tooth replacement.

The changed mouth contour also exposes you to biting problems. You may notice that your teeth have clamped down on your tongue or lips rather than on the food. It hurts, and it can be hard to avoid unless you chew carefully.

Vocal cords also age and fatigue more readily. Your voice will betray your age, particularly on the phone. If you are a singer or a member of a choral group, you may have to adjust your rehearsal time, or you may need professional help with voice retraining. Speech therapists can help.

Swallowing, a muscle effort coordinated with the throat, can become more difficult, sometimes allowing food particles to enter the trachea instead of the esophagus. This is a common cause of pneumonia. Chew more carefully. Swallow more slowly. Don't rush.

To Emphasize

1. Have your eyes checked.
2. If you notice any hearing loss, get a hearing test. Don't wait.
3. Don't blow your nose too hard. Sniff, don't blow.

CHAPTER 6

LUNGS
ANATOMY, FUNCTION, AND DISORDERS

By now, you are used to the idea that muscles get weaker with age. This applies as well to the muscles of respiration: the intercostal muscles between your ribs and the diaphragm. You are unable to take as deep a breath as before, nor can you force as strong a cough. These limitations alone are minor, but they become clinically important if you start having other problems.

Inhaled air passes down the trachea into ever narrower tubes until reaching the alveoli of the lungs. Gas exchange takes place there across a thin membrane—oxygen into the blood, carbon dioxide into the alveoli, from where carbon dioxide is exhaled. With aging, fewer alveoli remain intact, the respiratory tubes become stiffer, mucosal secretions diminish, and the fine cilia which transport foreign material back upwards become reduced. The lung has become more vulnerable to infection and gas exchange is impaired, but unless some superimposed problem exists or occurs, oxygen and carbon dioxide levels in the blood will remain normal throughout a long lifespan, less adaptable, but normal.

Pneumonia

Pneumonia is common and potentially very serious. Older patients, living alone, and simply believing they have a common cold with cough, may not want to go through the effort of seeking attention. It will soon pass, they think, and usually they are right, but it can also quickly worsen. Older individuals are sometimes found dead of pneumonia in their own homes, never having sought attention. Hence, if your cough worsens or lingers, or if you develop a fever, get immediate help.

I recall one such patient, a single, intelligent, healthy woman, age 72, whom I had seen infrequently over the years. One day I received a phone call from the coroner's office seeking information. Her neighbor in the building had heard her moving about earlier in the week, occasionally coughing, and knew she was home, but she did not respond to knocks on the door, and newspapers were piling up. Finally, the neighbor called the apartment manager, who entered the apartment and found her dead. He called the coroner. I had not seen her or heard from her for over one year. The autopsy showed pneumonia.

A similar circumstance arose with the husband of a friend. He was on a trip in Europe and developed an upper respiratory infection, which he self-treated in his hotel room, apparently resistant to getting help, or unclear how to obtain medical assistance. He was found dead, and the autopsy revealed pneumonia.

Corona viruses, or influenza viruses, or indeed any still unknown new viruses that might appear in epidemic form, give rise to the same sequence. Initially, an upper respiratory infection with cough appears, which can, though not necessarily does, lead to pneumonia and death. The elderly are particularly vulnerable.

When there is smoke, smog, or other air pollutants lingering in your environment, you are also more susceptible to respiratory infections. No wonder you often see people walking around with masks over their nose and mouth, even before the COVID-19 epidemic occurred. It is a good way to interrupt infections passing from one individual to another. Keep a few masks on hand at home in case you need them later.

Most of the time, however, a respiratory infection with cough, and perhaps mild blood-streaked sputum, will be due to a tracheal or bronchial viral inflammation, treatable with steam inhalations. If you do nothing else, it will require about two weeks to go away. If you take medications, they say it will take fourteen days. Antibiotics should almost never be used; they are much more likely to cause an allergic response or create antibiotic-resistant bacteria than they are likely to help you.

Emphysema and Other Chest Problems

Chronic obstructive pulmonary disease, also known as COPD, or emphysema, is common and progressively worsens with age. The usual cause is smoking, which leads to an inflammatory reaction in the bronchial mucosa, thereby reducing its cross-section area, narrowing the tube. As a consequence, air flow is obstructed, more in expiration than inspiration.

A similar process takes place with chronic asthma, which sometimes begins or worsens in older patients, in which case you will also hear pronounced wheezing. Inhalers and cortisone are often required.

Chronic obstruction to expiration will tend to produce expanding lungs, giving the chest a barrel-like look, a look enhanced by the presence of collapsed thoracic vertebral bodies. The appearance is of minor importance.

Your ribs, like bone elsewhere, become osteoporotic with age and prone to break. Even a light blow or a cough can fracture a rib. You will know you have done so because of the pain and the tenderness over the rib. The fracture will heal without treatment, but you may transiently want pain pills. However, if it hurts to breathe, make sure to take an occasional deep breath. You want your entire lung to be able to expand. If it cannot, areas of the lung will collapse, a condition called atelectasis, which reduces areas available for gas exchange. Preventing atelectasis also becomes important following surgery or anything leading to bed rest and reduced activity.

Occasionally, an intercostal muscle between two ribs will sustain a tear, often in the mid-thoracic area posteriorly, usually due to a cough or a straining movement. There is discomfort in the area, and sometimes a small lump can be felt over the muscle. Massaging the area at home usually suffices for treatment.

To Emphasize

1. Most colds with cough do not require antibiotics.
2. Steam inhalations are good cough suppressants.
3. Don't smoke anything.

CHAPTER 7

HEART AND BLOOD VESSELS
ANATOMY, FUNCTION, AND DISEASE

The heart is a muscle, and when it contracts, it pushes blood through the arteries to the capillaries. It pumps less well with age, and some heart muscle gets replaced with fibrous tissue. Fibrous tissue also replaces some elastic tissue in the arterial walls so that both heart and arteries become stiffer. A stiffer artery is a less distensible one; hence, blood pressure increases with aging. Nonetheless, if nothing else happens, this system will continue operating through a lifetime. But something, sooner or later, will always happen, either to the blood vessels, the valves within the heart, or the heart muscle itself.

Artery Disorders and Hypertension

Arteriosclerosis is the term used to denote stiffening or hardening of the arterial wall. Old enough, and you will have it. It increases with age, and with age it becomes complicated by the addition of cholesterol plaques and calcium in the inner lining of the artery wall, a condition called atherosclerosis.

If a clot should form on the plaque, it can block the artery entirely. When this occurs in the heart, it is called a coronary thrombosis, which is the usual cause of what is known as a heart attack.

Cholesterol depositions within arterial walls can also break away and settle in a smaller artery, blocking it from that point onward. These cholesterol particles, which also contain blood clot parts, are called emboli.

Risk factors for developing plaques are:

1. Genetic predisposition
2. Smoking
3. Diabetes
4. Obesity
5. Cholesterol or lipid abnormalities
6. High blood pressure

High blood pressure is very common in adults. It is usually due to essential hypertension. Hypertension can also be due to uncommon causes, such as hormonal abnormalities. The word "essential" simply refers to the fact that all its causes are unknown, but a strong heart pulse against a slightly rigid arterial wall is one unifying factor. Treatment begun earlier will almost always have to be continued as you enter older decades, because the arterial wall continually stiffens with age. Ultimately, however, your heart might beat less forcibly and allow a reduction or even a discontinuance of medication.

How to treat hypertension is always age-dependent. A stable blood pressure of 140/90 in a 25-year-old is worrisome because it will remain elevated for many years, and worsen. It needs treatment. Even a slightly higher blood pressure which arises in an 85-year-old though, may not need treatment, for it will operate over a much shorter period, and medication problems may outweigh benefits.

With time, arterial circulation worsens in everyone. The arterial lumen becomes reduced, and the heart pumps less strongly. As a result, blood flow to organs, muscles, and tissues becomes diminished, and if severe enough, symptoms result. A characteristic example occurs in the arteries to the legs. There is enough circulation at rest, but with increased walking, calf pain can occur, a condition called claudication.

Diminished arterial circulation in the legs also causes visible changes in the feet. They might be paler on elevation, and duskier on lowering them. Nails are less well nourished and become thicker. Skin breaks heal more slowly, particularly over the shin, an area notoriously known for poor healing because arterial flow to the feet descends mainly down the back of the leg. This is unfortunate, as it is the front of the leg, the shin, which is the area that gets readily bumped, causing elderly skin to tear.

Vein Disorders

Blood returns from the capillaries to the heart in veins, usually working against gravity. What propels the blood is a slight push from the contracting heart, and from muscular contractions squeezing the blood upwards. There are thin valves within the veins, holding the blood in place, or rather preventing it from flowing backwards.

Over many years, gravity begins to win. The valves can no longer retard all the back flow. Veins become more prominent, even varicose in some people. Venous flow slows and pressure within the veins increases, causing fluid and other blood elements to leave the circulation. Swelling, discoloration, and reduced vitality of the underlying tissues result. Even minor trauma can then cause ulceration of the skin, which remains difficult to treat. The inside of the ankle is a characteristic site. Treatment involves keeping the ulcer clean and reducing swelling with elevation and pressure dressings.

Clots can arise in superficial veins, both in the legs and in the arms. They are visible, almost never migrate, and are best treated by applying warm compresses over the site.

Clots in deep veins, on the other hand, always cause problems. They are generally invisible. Often they block venous return enough to cause swelling. They can also break off and pass up the entire venous system, through the right atrium into the right ventricle, and lodge in a major pulmonary artery, a condition called a pulmonary embolus. It is a frequent cause of death in postoperative patients.

There are three principle risk factors for the development of these deep venous thrombi:

1. Blood clotting abnormalities which may have been unknown
2. Trauma to a venous wall, providing an irregular surface on which a clot can form
3. Stasis, hence marked slowing of venous flow, favoring clotting

Surgery and postoperative immobility are known precursors, but anything that forces bed rest or prolonged sitting, such as in an airplane, is suspect. Since these clots are often asymptomatic, it is up to the patient to keep leg muscles pumping and to elevate legs as often as feasible in order to assist venous return. One consult I recall was a woman in her early 50s, suspected of having a heart attack because of chest heaviness. It is not a common diagnosis in women in that age group, and further questioning revealed she had been experiencing shortness of breath beginning after a recent four-hour airplane flight. What she turned out to have were pulmonary emboli, requiring urgent anticoagulant therapy to cure her. Sitting in the plane without moving enough caused a clot to form in a large leg vein, from which smaller clots broke off and flowed to her lungs. Had the large clot broken away, she would have died.

Heart Valve Disorders

Heart valves open to enable blood to pass through, and then they close to prevent the blood from flowing back. Unless there have been congenital abnormalities, or early rheumatic disorders, they function normally well into old age. But you know by now that after many years of use, things can happen. Valvular problems can arise. Why in some people more than others is not always clear.

Presumably a genetic predisposition has led to changes on the valve surface. The valve becomes distorted, favoring deposition of calcium and cholesterol, further damaging the valve and partially blocking blood flow.

Stenosis of the aortic valve (the valve between the left ventricle and the aorta) is the classic common example. Two things happen: Not enough blood gets through to the coronary artery or to the brain, causing faintness; and the blocked valve increases pressure backwards into the lung, causing shortness of breath and heaviness. If you notice any of these symptoms, get medical help.

Just because a valve leaks, however, does not necessarily mean treatment is required. Ultrasound studies of the valves in older patients routinely demonstrate abnormalities, for which treatment is often not needed, or perhaps even unavailable. Yet, an abnormal valve is not as good as a normal one, and any valvular change can be one of several contributions to the shortness of breath, which you will begin to experience with exertion.

Heart Rhythm Disorders

An electrical discharge starting from a cluster of small cells on the external surface of the heart at the junction of the right atrium and superior vena cava, and then spreading down the heart, initiates each normal heart contraction. Fibrosis can disrupt this electrical circuitry, as can a myocardial infarction. Abnormal rhythms result, too fast, too slow, or irregular, which patients usually notice. If you do notice such a pulse change and also have faintness, chest pain, or shortness of breath, you should get medical help promptly. These symptoms also can occur with a myocardial infarction, i.e., a heart attack.

You have heard of pacemakers. When the electrical impulse is too slow, a pacemaker (a battery-driven electrical impulse inserted under the skin and attached to the heart) will provide the electrical impulse to initiate a contraction.

And you've heard of blood thinners or anticoagulants. When are they used in heart disease? The most common, sustained, troublesome, heart rhythm disturbance, by far, is atrial fibrillation, an irregularly initiated rapid heartbeat that disallows complete contraction of the entire left atrium, enabling blood to pool. With pooling or stasis, there is an increased chance of blood clots, which then can pass into the arterial circulation, causing, among other problems, a stroke. Anticoagulants retard, but may not entirely eliminate this clotting potential, one reason why cardiologists might try to eliminate fibrillation by other means.

Heart Attack and Heart Failure

Heart attacks result from an abrupt loss of blood supply to a part of the heart wall, usually from a blocked coronary artery. The heart muscle now suddenly deprived of blood can no longer pump normally. Although most patients will survive, the degree of survival will depend upon how much heart muscle is involved. Preventing a heart attack requires reducing or eliminating the risk factors for plaque formation already mentioned above: smoking, hypertension, high cholesterol, diabetes, and obesity.

If there is a strong family history for heart attacks, you might also consider becoming a blood donor, something you can do into your 80s, for there is an unpublished suggestion that thinning blood, thus increasing blood flow, might retard clot formation.

The idea arose out of the fact that premenopausal women who maintain regular menses are far less likely than men to have a heart attack. But once past menopause, they are no longer protected. Why this difference was never clearly established.

One consequence of regular menses is a lower red blood cell count when compared to men, hence thinner blood. One other way to obtain a lower red blood cell count and thinner blood is to donate blood at a blood bank. Studies I performed years ago indicated that men with known coronary atherosclerotic disease had been far less likely to donate blood, a suggestion, not a proof, that blood donation might benefit coronary-prone patients.

The older the heart, the less well it functions, and if there has been enough additional damage due to heart attacks, hypertension, or a rare heart muscle disease, congestive heart failure ensues. One of two conditions, or both, explain this heart failure. Either not enough blood is being pumped out (systolic dysfunction), or the heart muscle has become too fibrotic and cannot relax enough to contain all the blood accumulating (diastolic dysfunction). Ultimately, symptoms arise: fatigue, shortness of breath, swollen feet, or a swollen abdomen. Diuretics help. Yet congestive heart failure is one common cause of death.

To Emphasize

1. New onset chest pain requires evaluation.
2. Regular exercise to increase your heart rate is healthy at every age.
3. Treat all swollen ankles with elevation. Add diuretics, if needed.

CHAPTER 8

GASTROINTESTINAL TRACT

"WHEN YOU ARE 20 YEARS OLD, YOU TALK ABOUT THE DATE YOU HAD THE NIGHT BEFORE. WHEN YOU ARE 50 YEARS OLD, YOU TALK ABOUT THE DINNER YOU HAD THE NIGHT BEFORE. AND WHEN YOU ARE 80, YOU TALK ABOUT THE BOWEL MOVEMENT YOU HAD THE THE NIGHT BEFORE."

SO BEGAN THE ONE AND ONLY GERIATRIC LECTURE I HAD IN MEDICAL SCHOOL. SINCE THEN THE GERIATRIC CURRICULUM HAS GREATLY EXPANDED.

Esophagus - Swallowing Problems

Nutrients enter the esophagus with the help of a coordinated muscular activity propelling material from throat to stomach via an opening at the gastroesophageal junction. It will be impaired if muscular contractions become uncoordinated due to aging, if obstruction develops, or when stomach acids regurgitate too often and inflame the lower esophagus. Difficulty swallowing results, which, if persistent, requires medical attention.

Acid regurgitation also causes heartburn, characteristically 30 to 60 minutes after meals, or upon reclining, or after activities requiring prolonged bending over. It is best managed by avoiding caffeine, alcohol, or heavy meals close to bedtime, and treating any symptoms by sitting up, drinking water, and swallowing your saliva (which is alkaline). Antacids provide more reliable relief, and Tums, for example, also provides some calcium. Nonetheless, do not use antacids daily; stomach acids have an important role in preventing bacterial growth, and antacids will interfere with this protection.

Make sure you chew food enough so that the small particles pass more readily. If you are still having trouble swallowing, try lifting your head higher and throwing your shoulders back. It will straighten your esophagus and enable easier swallowing. In the unusual event that a piece of meat gets stuck in your lower esophagus, no matter what you have heard, do not use meat tenderizer. It will damage the esophageal lining. You can try soda water, hoping the bubbles will do something, but usually you will have to go to an Emergency Room for endoscopy.

A much more serious swallowing accident occurs when a piece of meat, instead of entering the esophagus, enters the trachea or larynx and obstructs. The elderly and denture wearers are particularly at risk. You cannot breathe, cough, or talk, and you have three to four minutes to get rid of the obstruction. If others are around, point to your neck and attract attention for help. You want someone to perform a Heimlich maneuver, by standing behind you and pushing upwards over your epigastrium (upper abdomen) while you are bent forward. If you are alone, you will have to do the pushing, by leaning over a chair.

If acid regurgitates more readily into your esophagus, it can even enter your pharynx, trachea, or larynx during sleep. One sign that this may be occurring is a brackish taste, unexplained cough, or morning hoarseness. Sleeping with your chest about 30 degrees upright should prevent most symptoms.

Stomach and Small Intestines

In the stomach and small intestines, nutrient mixing and absorption take place, essentially unhindered by aging. If you happen to have developed an intolerance to some food, it would usually result in diarrhea. Diarrhea is also caused by food poisoning from bacterial contamination of something you have just eaten. This can occur at any age and is often accompanied by vomiting. Your body reacts by adding large amounts of fluid to the intestinal tract, thereby producing diarrhea, which ordinarily will only last a few hours. Nonetheless, it will take two to three days for your intestines to recover. During this time, stay with simple foods, clear liquids, and no milk products, for they will be absorbed poorly during this recovery phase. You will not need medications.

With aging, the stomach produces less acid, and peptic ulcers become uncommon, but cancers occur more frequently. The mean age of stomach cancer at diagnosis is 63 years; hence, it can be a geriatric problem, first manifested by new onset gastric symptoms that persist. Endoscopy will be indicated.

Indigestion and abdominal discomfort are common, but, ordinarily, they are transient. Simply by modifying your diet, for example to clear liquids, you will get better. If low-grade indigestion persists, try omitting milk products or gluten. Avoid aspirin or any NSAID (non-steroidal anti-inflammatory drug), both of which produce shallow stomach ulcers in many individuals. If abdominal pain persists, you worry about appendicitis. One test you can do on yourself at home is to bend from the waist and push deeply into your right lower abdomen. If it hurts, you probably have appendicitis. If it hurts on the left side, you could have diverticulitis, a colon problem treated with antibiotics.

Colon and Rectum

Constipation is a common geriatric problem, sometimes so severe that fecal impaction occurs, necessitating digital removal of feces from the rectum. You may also have to give yourself enemas. You can do all this, but it's not easy.

Normal colonic transit time is up to 35 hours, so not having a bowel movement for that long may not be abnormal. Plenty of fluid enters the colon, but only about 10% passes out. If there is too little water in the feces, hard and difficult-to-eliminate bowel movements occur. To prevent constipation, drink more water and eat more dietary fiber, up to 30 grams daily may be required. It is largely unabsorbed and hence provides water-containing bulk to your stools. Nonetheless, you may occasionally or even frequently have to add over-the-counter laxatives.

Constipation with straining also leads to diverticula, which are little pouches in the colon mucosa. They become increasingly common with age; indeed half of individuals over age 80 will have diverticula. Although often asymptomatic, complications arise that include bleeding, inflammation, and perforation, all calling for medical attention.

Colorectal cancer screening by colonoscopy is usually confined to the 50- to 75-year age group, often performed every 10 years unless known polyps or family history prompt more frequent study. Colonoscopy is cumbersome, particularly for the elderly, hence in many cases replaceable by less sensitive testing for occult fecal blood.

If you see streaks of blood on toilet paper, it is almost always due to anal hemorrhoids and not from cancer. Nonetheless, if the problem continues, or if you have noticed a persisting change in your bowel habits, seek help. Colorectal cancers are common; they are the second leading cause of death due to malignancy in the United States.

If you have anal itching, never wash the area with soap, which is likely irritating the area and causing the itch. Fecal matter, urine, dirt, mud, and most items striking your skin will all be water soluble. A shower or a bath without soap is all that is usually required.

Abdominal wall hernias also occur with increasing frequency with aging, most usually in the inguinal area. They are due to muscle weakness in isolated areas, at which increased intra-abdominal pressure from coughing or straining will push out hernias. They rarely require surgery unless large, but they may cause occasional discomfort.

Liver and Gall Bladder

You can live a lifetime without knowing you have a gallbladder, and it can be removed without interfering with lifespan. Indeed, it should be removed if you have symptoms. Gallstones are common, and when they block the flow of bile, you will have pain in the right upper part of your abdomen, as well as oftentimes fever. You can worsen quickly; hence, no matter your age, get help. The oldest patient I saw needing gallbladder surgery was 98.

All the venous blood from the intestinal tract passes via the portal vein through the liver, which then removes toxins. A liver too damaged to function well, usually because of alcoholism or prior hepatitis, needs replacement with transplant, an option not available to the elderly because of a scant supply of donor livers. On the other hand, aging alone will not lead to liver failure, but it does cause a lessened ability to detoxify, one reason why drug dosages often need modification when you age.

To Emphasize

1. Avoid daily antacids or NSAIDS.
2. Severe or continuing abdominal pain requires medical attention.
3. If constipated, add more fiber to your diet.

CHAPTER 9

GENITOURINARY SYSTEM IN MEN AND WOMEN

The kidneys filter blood to make urine. With aging, many kidney cells stop functioning well, a process hastened by hypertension or diabetes. Nonetheless, the great majority of individuals retain adequate function throughout their lives. The dosage of any drugs excreted through the kidney, however, will need lowering in the elderly because of a reduced capacity to excrete the drug.

What happens when kidneys fail? Some fifty years ago, there was no treatment. Toxins accumulated, and all patients died. Now there are transplants and dialysis. There are not enough transplantable kidneys available; hence, transplanting in the elderly is usually not an option. But patients can be maintained on dialysis well into their 90s. It is a definite handicap and requires access to a dialysis unit three times a week, but patients can stay alive and near-normal as long as dialysis continues.

Incontinence

The urinary bladder wall is a muscle, the detrusor, which, on contracting, excretes urine through the urethra. When the bladder fills with urine, nerves in the bladder wall sense this stretching and send impulses to the brain that it is time to urinate voluntarily. You

44

can suppress these impulses, but they will recur, and ultimately you must urinate.

The older you are, the harder to ignore the urge to urinate, and you may have involuntary partial bladder contractions causing urinary leakage, a condition called urge incontinence. A lifetime of conditioned reflexes may also cause hard-to-suppress urges to urinate. For example, just putting a key into your front door on coming home can stimulate a strong urge to urinate. Leakage is embarrassing and a nuisance. Steps to prevent urge incontinence include trying to hold a full bladder while at home, and then stopping urine flow in midstream. By continuing to exercise the muscles stopping flow, you may find you have gained better control. You can sense what these muscles are when you stop urine flow a few times. Basically, it involves tightening pelvic muscles, something you can easily do on occasion each day. Also try to anticipate future needs to urinate in order to avoid being caught unawares.

A different type of incontinence is that leakage which occurs on coughing or on increasing intra-abdominal pressure, for example, when lifting. Such activities can overcome the pelvic floor sphincter muscles that keep urine in your bladder. Women who have had vaginal deliveries or pelvic surgery are particularly at risk for this so-called stress incontinence. Treatment begins with pelvic floor exercises, done by squeezing together pelvic muscles while thrusting the pelvis forward, a maneuver popularly known as a Kegel exercise. You must perform it frequently in order to have any improvement.

Prostate

Contrary to the usual rule that organs get smaller with age, the prostate enlarges, a process called benign prostatic hyperplasia. It presents in over 90% of men aged 80 years or above. This hyperplasia may frequently also contain some malignant cells. In fact, autopsies reveal cancer in some two thirds of men age 80 to 90 years. But most men will die with these cancer cells and not because of them. Nonetheless, prostate cancer is a relatively common cause of death.

How to distinguish which prostate cancers require treatment is a problem for a urologist. The determinations are ordinarily based on PSA studies (blood tests), rectal examination, and biopsies obtained through the rectum. While all such studies are important in men up to the age of 70 or so, particularly in the presence of a family history for prostate cancer, routine screening after age 70 is rarely indicated, in part because screening has side-effects, and in part because any cancers found are usually slow growing. If faster growing, treatment can always be started later with little or no loss of efficacy.

Prostate growth with aging partially encircles the upper urethra and also bulks into the bladder. As a result, you may have to strain somewhat to pass urine or to initiate urination. You will also see a thinner urinary stream and might sense that bladder emptying is incomplete. Incomplete emptying often leads to an urge to urinate again, shortly after having just done so.

If urinary obstruction is severe enough, you will have to consult a urologist. There are surgical treatment options.

Impotence or Erectile Dysfunction

Questions regarding sexual organ function occur at almost any age, though usually asked reluctantly. Patients who consulted me with sexual questions were, understandably, practically exclusively men, women surely being more comfortable having any such discussion with their gynecologist.

A few years ago, I examined a 74-year-old lifelong bachelor, living alone in a downtown apartment building, who came for a routine examination. He was a worrier but had no symptoms. Under such circumstances, physical examination tends to disclose no pertinent abnormalities, and such indeed was the case.

I needed to reassure him of his good general health, and of ways to maintain it. Since single older men are prone to depression and suicide, our conversation turned to the notion that with so many single older women in his neighborhood, marriage could offer advantages. I must admit I was also curious how this confirmed bachelor would respond to that suggestion. "Who would want me?" he replied, "I'm impudent."

Although impudence in this age group would probably test a marriage more than impotence, the delightful malapropism indicates that impotence or erectile dysfunction (ED) was at least on his mind, problem or not.

Erectile dysfunction can be partial or complete, and is age dependent. It is also influenced by psychological, social, and cultural factors; by marital history; by prior sexual habits; and by overall health of both patient and partner. About 70% of men over age 65, nonetheless, are sexually active to some degree, a number that drops progressively decade by decade thereafter, even when libido, sexual interests, arousal, and erections might still occur. There are no good studies, however, about any of these numbers, nor are there particularly good studies about the overall efficacy of drugs such as Viagra to treat ED.

With aging, the testes become smaller, and testosterone secretion diminishes. Whether this partial testosterone deficiency has any important clinical sequel is unclear, or at least any consequence which should be treated. Testosterone replacement is cumbersome and of no proven benefit. It has side effects. Avoid it.

Gynecology

After menopause, ovaries shrink and most of their hormonal activity diminishes. The vagina becomes dry due to decreased secretions and narrowed by fibrosis and atrophy. Partial uterine prolapse can occur without the person knowing it. All of these problems worsen with progressing age, and they can make intercourse painful or even impossible. Despite reduced estrogen secretions, systemic hormone replacement therapy is controversial. It will usually cause more problems than it will solve.

Ovarian and uterine cancers become more frequent. Cervical cancers become less frequent, and Pap tests, which screen for cervical cancers, are usually no longer needed above the age of 65.

Most ovarian growths are benign, but all need evaluating. They are often asymptomatic until they grow larger, when rather nonspecific symptoms might occur. Unfortunately, about 75% of ovarian cancers are diagnosed with advanced disease, hence reducing potential survival, which might otherwise be favorable with an earlier diagnosis.

Vaginal bleeding, an indicator of uterine cancer, always requires investigation, even if it only occurs once, whether painless or not. Many causes are benign, but not all.

With advanced age, pelvic organ prolapse of urinary bladder or rectum into the vagina can occur and is seen more commonly in multiparous or obese women. It can be small and asymptomatic, but it may also produce a sensation of a vaginal bulge or interfere with bowel movements or urination. The only cure for symptomatic prolapse is corrective surgery.

The well-known Kinsey reports from the 1950s, which revealed the sexual habits of Americans, largely concerned an age group 45 and under. There was no mention of any sexual function studies above the age of 60. Yet sexual activity clearly continues, and sexual thoughts, libido, and arousal occur, at least into the 80s. However, since perhaps the majority of older women, at least above the age of 75, live without spouses or partners, sexual activity becomes difficult, and masturbation may be the primary outlet for orgasmic activity. How often, how easily this occurs are areas not documented. There are no studies, nor necessarily need there be. Intimacy, connecting with others, though, remains important at any age.

To Emphasize

1. Pelvic floor exercises will reduce incontinence.
2. Blood in urine or in vaginal secretions is abnormal.
3. Almost all sexual activity is normal.

CHAPTER 10

ENDOCRINE DISORDERS AND DIABETES

Endocrine problems occur fairly frequently throughout life, most secondary to reduced rather than increased hormonal secretions. The major geriatric endocrine diagnosis, diabetes, is one that becomes increasingly more common with advancing age. It is caused by reduced secretion of insulin or reduced sensitivity to the insulin secreted.

Insulin is secreted from a small part of the pancreas, and disorders of insulin secretion cause diabetes Type 2, also known as adult diabetes. It affects over 10% of older patients. Insulin receptors have become less sensitive to rising glucose levels, causing delays in insulin secretion. Obesity and family history are risk factors. The earliest sign, a mild elevation of blood glucose, called pre-diabetes, is asymptomatic. In fact, overt diabetes mellitus, where blood glucose determinations are consistently increased, is also often asymptomatic, first recognized in a routine examination or in conjunction with the evaluation of another disease.

When diabetes arises abruptly and unexpectedly in an older patient, it could be due to pancreatic cancer, which had begun to invade adjacent insulin-producing cells.

I had one such patient. He actually belonged to a medical family, which, in practice, often results in such patients going directly to the specialist they deem most appropriate for the complaint. He had very vague but annoying abdominal discomfort and sought a gastroenterologist, who found no abdominal abnormality. By the time I saw him a few weeks later, he had developed insulin-dependent diabetes. An abdominal CT scan revealed pancreatic cancer. Unfortunately, even with an early diagnosis, pancreatic cancer is almost always uniformly fatal. With chemotherapy and remissions, he was able to live another five years.

It is exceedingly important to recognize diabetes, though, because elevated blood sugars will hasten the development of vascular, heart, kidney, and neurological diseases. Patients improve with a diet, exercise program, and weight control. Physicians might also add medications, and all patients will require ongoing surveillance with blood testing.

The only other relatively common, or at least not to be missed geriatric endocrine disorder, is low thyroid. It is often manifested by low energy states, but it can also be asymptomatic. A simple test will make the diagnosis. Treatment is easy and involves the replacement of thyroid hormone.

Neither parathyroid nor adrenal glands have specific geriatric syndromes. Although touted to increase energy and well-being in older patients, there is no indication for pituitary manipulation or for the injection of human growth hormone.

To Emphasize

1. Exercise reduces blood glucose.
2. Obtain an occasional diabetes test.
3. If overweight, losing pounds is hard but helpful.

CHAPTER 11

BRAIN AND NERVOUS SYSTEM

Even though you are older, have lost neurons, have become physically less adept, and react more slowly, your basic understanding of life, your perceptions, your wisdoms, your expressions, your overall memory can remain intact a lifetime. Yet something known as benign forgetfulness of aging does occur. After all, by the time you are 80, your brain is filled with about twice as many impressions as it was when you were 40. It is no wonder, therefore, that you may not immediately recall someone's name or remember the plot of a movie you saw one week earlier. Don't panic. The reason you can remember many eighth-grade classmates' names is that you store that information in a brain far less cluttered than the one you currently have. If you can't remember something, but know what it is you can't remember, it is rarely the beginning of dementia. It's an important point that bears repeating. IF YOU CAN'T REMEMBER SOMETHING, BUT KNOW WHAT IT IS YOU CAN'T REMEMBER, IT IS RARELY THE BEGINNING OF DEMENTIA.

Dementia - Memory Loss

Dementia is a common, serious problem. The World Health Organization expects the number of people suffering from dementia to increase by a factor of three before the year 2050. In some patients it rapidly progresses over one to two years, but more usually there is a long cognitive decline over five to ten years. In its milder, early stages, it may only be noticed by a close friend or family member who sees that the person has already forgotten something just discussed.

While distant memories remain intact, a common feature of dementia is loss of recent memory. It is something you can test by asking the individual to try to remember three words, for example, blue, pencil, book. Once these three words are successfully repeated, go on to other activities, and then periodically afterwards, ask the person to name those three items again. If the person can recall those items as well as you, there is no dementia, but most Alzheimer patients have largely forgotten them within thirty minutes. Another simple test of how well someone can integrate information is to ask them to draw a clock with a specific time, for example, 3:20. Dementia patients usually cannot do this correctly. There are more sophisticated studies available, but the results of these rarely aid patient management. Once a diagnosis of dementia is made in a licensed driver, the Department of Motor Vehicles must be notified.

Alzheimer's Disease

Most dementias by far are due to Alzheimer's disease, a disorder characterized pathologically by the presence of amyloid plaques and neurofibrillary tangles in the brain. Like almost everything else affecting patients, there may be a genetic predisposition. No other specific cause has yet been identified. Other rarer neurodegenerative disorders can also lead to dementia, as can brains damaged by cerebrovascular disorders, head trauma, or Parkinson's disease.

The name Alzheimer derived from the name of Alois Alzheimer, a German pathologist, who in 1907 described the brain changes he noticed at autopsy on a 57-year-old woman who had died with dementia. The disorder seemed to be uncommon, but because it occurred in middle age, it became known as pre-senile dementia.

Much later, when autopsies performed on elderly patients with dementia showed the same neurofibrillary tangles that Alzheimer had described, it became recognized that the disease was the same, euphemistically called "old-timer's disease" for those with trouble pronouncing a German name. In advanced, end-stage Alzheimer's disease, in which many neurons have died and disappeared in the cerebral cortex (presumably because the fibrillary tangles interfered with neuronal health), the resultant cerebral atrophy and loss of function can become extreme.

However, with almost-mute patients lying in a bed, unaware of their surroundings, there might be pockets of understanding. A very recent documentary film showed such a patient, bedridden, not responding to his surroundings, who, when headphones were placed over his ears sounding music from his youth, responded with a joyful expression and an attempted motion to keep time with the music. The same response was observed in a former member of a chorus when his old chorus music companions came to his bedside and sang some of the songs they had all known.

Clearly, even in advanced cases, some brain function is left. A response occurs, and the question arises whether musical stimulation should become a form of therapy for such patients. At least, it seems to create joy.

Brain tumors, thyroid disorders, B12 deficiency, HIV diseases, severe depressions, and various medications (particularly acetylcholine inhibitors) can sometimes present with what appears to be dementia. Since they offer treatment in what is otherwise an untreatable dementia, these conditions must be ruled out.

Alzheimer Treatment

Because there are so many patients with dementia, pharmaceutical companies continue to seek treatments. Yet none so far have really helped. There are also claims, not proofs, that some drugs seem to slow the progression of Alzheimer's disease, but simply slowing progression of a very disabling disorder, unless begun very early, is of no long-term benefit, and these drugs are expensive. They also can have serious side effects.

Numerous studies have suggested that links between physical fitness and brain health may retard the development of Alzheimer's disease. Therefore, exercise is good therapy. Keeping the mind engaged is also important. Book clubs, playing bridge, discussion groups, volunteering for a political candidate, learning a new language, and all such activities might help. An interesting technique is to have the patient begin a favorite book, a mystery, a biography, or a novel, and read a chapter each night, thereby needing to remember in order to continue the reading. There is no hard evidence that these activities really help, but like physical exercise, they might, and they can't hurt. Remember: Use it or lose it applies to the mind as well as to the body.

In early dementia, the burden of care usually falls on a spouse, a partner, or another family member living with the patient. But a different kind of problem arises when the individual is still living independently. He or she will soon need assistance, usually through some kind of guardianship in order to supervise financial, residential, and healthcare issues. If family is unavailable, social services can help, as can legal aids. Don't wait too long to make any needed arrangements. It is much easier early on when the patient still has understanding and can remain part of the solution.

Once someone presents with established dementia, adequate help becomes a necessity. Try to make sure that the patient maintains dignity and agency. Have the patient make out a schedule of activities or a list of where items are stored. Even when you know that he or she cannot readily respond to a question, allow them to try. Asking "What would you like for lunch?" or "Where should I place this vase?" involves the patient, who otherwise would have no reason to think. It is a very common error to answer in place of patients, often to save them possible anguish, or to speed things along, but nonetheless, try not to intervene. Know, also, that the calmer the setting, the less disruptive the living conditions, the less the confusion.

When dementia has progressed to a degree so that patients are unaware of their surroundings, a different concern arises. If patients are physically strong and leave the house or living quarters, they will get lost. They need protection. Many patients, though, are weak or bedridden, bewildered, and often unable to feed themselves. These essentially ethical problems need resolutions from the beginning, usually in conjunction with a council of family members and caregivers. Almost all, if not all, medications should have long ago been stopped if the patient is incapacitated and unaware of surroundings. Surprisingly, many medications are still being given. Don't be afraid to ask why.

Also inquire about "Do not resuscitate orders" (DNR), which are appropriate for demented patients. Make sure that all care-givers recognize what DNR means. Similarly, make sure that care-givers know that such patients should never be transferred to hospital emergency rooms. Unaware of their surroundings, these patients are much better off managed where they are living.

With a population becoming increasingly older, dementia problems will increase. Most have causes still unidentified, and none have good pharmaceutical treatments. They will remain a burden to families and to society for the foreseeable future. But the brain, like other organs, can repair, at least partially, an injury. Hence, opening previously unused neural pathways by learning new tasks might bypass some of the areas of brain disease. It's worth trying since new neural routing could create a better functioning brain.

Parkinson's Disease

Parkinson's disease is the most common serious movement disorder neurologists confront. Although it usually begins between ages 45 to 65, it may be difficult to diagnose at its onset. Yet it develops slowly enough and is common enough that it becomes unmistakable with aging or in the elderly. Of unknown cause, this degenerative disorder involving a part of the brain called the extra-pyramidal system is relentlessly progressive, in some patients slower, in others faster. Medications stall its progress, and home movement exercises help reduce the accompanying muscular rigidity. Physiotherapists can define what exercises are beneficial.

The pill-rolling hand tremor and a relatively immobile face, combined with slowness of voluntary movements and a reduction of automatic movements, such as arm swinging while walking, are cardinal features of Parkinson's disease. In time, the disease becomes a frequent cause or a contributor to a patient's death, often in their sixth to eighth decade.

About ten percent of so-called Parkinson patients do not have Parkinson's disease at all. The signs and symptoms of the disease are there because of drug side effects, most notably from antidepressants or antipsychotic drugs. Often these arise soon after treatment has begun, or after increasing the dose of the causative drug. Unlike Parkinson's disease, which progresses slowly, drug-induced Parkinsonism advances more quickly, over weeks to months, but it also tends to disappear quickly over one to two months once the offending drug has been removed.

Hand tremors related to aging are relatively common and should not be confused with Parkinson tremors. They are less coarse, appear on use, are visible but minor, and often become reduced with alcohol.

Stroke

Strokes are due to an abrupt loss of blood supply to a part of the brain due to a thrombus or, less often, due to an acute hemorrhage into the brain through a break in a cerebral artery wall—-hence the term cerebrovascular accident (CVA). Characteristically, one side of the body has a partial or a total paralysis. Speech may also be affected.

Transient ischemia attacks (TIAs) often herald a later stroke.

As the name implies, they represent fleeting neurologic or visual loss. They are due to a temporary blockage of a smaller cerebral artery from a thrombus, which has spontaneously dissolved. Yet they indicate that a serious potential problem exists. Hence, when they arise, they require urgent investigation. They are usually due to clots migrating to the brain from the heart or from a carotid artery. From which of those two sites needs to be identified. The treatments differ.

Once a stroke has occurred, hospitalization as soon as possible is necessary, for early treatment might reduce subsequent neurologic deficit.

Although stroke is a leading cause of death, most patients survive the initial stroke. Prognosis is better with strokes not involving hemorrhage. Having had one stroke, though, makes a patient slightly more vulnerable to another one. Because the underlying causes of this brain disorder reside in the cardiovascular system, therapies for prevention are cardiovascular.

Physical therapy (PT) is an important part of stroke treatment. At first, passive movement of any paralyzed limbs will minimize the common occurrence that these limbs become increasingly contracted. Thereafter, as patients become more alert and able to follow instructions, PT involves active exercise. Occupational therapists can help with motor skills, and speech therapists with talking. When motor deficits persist, physical therapists can organize devices such as leg braces or proper chairs to enable increasing activity. Improvement will ordinarily take place, but it may take months or years.

Headache, Nerves, and Myalgia

Headaches are common in our society, but the only one specifically linked with aging is due to giant cell arteritis, which is often accompanied by muscle aches and malaise. Physical examination usually reveals tenderness over the temporal arteries, which are located in front of the ears. Early diagnosis is important, for blindness can occur if this immune disorder is not recognized and treated.

There are many other causes for headache, some of which will need evaluation, indeed always when brain function seems impaired. Be especially concerned if a head injury had occurred days or weeks earlier. Under such circumstances, there might be an expanding blood clot on the brain surface needing evacuation. Older patients, particularly, might not remember a recent fall or blow on the head.

Peripheral nerves function near normal a lifetime, but aging changes will reduce function, particularly in the nerves furthest from the brain—those to the feet. Impulses between the brain and distant nerves become compromised. Walking becomes less nimble. Neuropathies occur, deep tendon reflexes become lost, and, if sensations become diminished, you might not feel a pebble in your shoe. Should you then develop an ulcer on your sole, it will be hard to treat. Examine your feet often to catch any problems at their onset.

Aging-induced peripheral neuropathy has no effective medication or therapy, so don't waste money on advertised claims. On the other hand, there are conditions which can cause peripheral neuropathy and must be eliminated as possible sources. These include B1 deficiency, B12 deficiency, alcohol excess, and diabetes.

In some patients, the neuropathy causes a burning pain in the toe tips or soles. It makes no sense that this symptom should be particularly worse at night, but it often is, perhaps because there is nothing else to distract you then. Walking and foot use also reduce toe symptoms, something, though, you prefer to avoid at bedtime. If the discomfort interferes with sleep, sometimes applying 5% lidocaine cream in the area might help. Neurologists use nerve conduction studies to verify the diagnosis, but whether any drug therapy helps is unclear.

Another condition of nerve and muscle seen occasionally in older patients is polymyalgia rheumatica (PMR), which presents with such non-specific symptoms as body aching, vague malaise, and low energy. It is important to recognize and easy to diagnose with a simple blood test (an elevated sedimentation rate). It is easy to treat with low dose prednisone. Inasmuch as I saw several cases in my own private practice, this immune disorder may actually be quite common.

To Emphasize

1. Physical activity is good for mental activity.
2. No matter what your age, continue learning.
3. New onset mental confusion requires investigation.

CHAPTER 12

PSYCHIATRIC PROBLEMS

"LIFE IS PARADISE —- HIDDEN IN EACH
ONE OF US."

FYODOR DOSTOEVSKY

Younger patients have somewhat different psychiatric concerns than older patients. They are more troubled with stress and adjustment disorders, chronic pain syndromes, psychosexual worries, post-traumatic issues. They have more anxieties and neuroses.

Older patients, simply by virtue of being older and more experienced, may have been able to resolve some of the situational difficulties that troubled younger patients. But they have different problems, often in the realm of mood disorders, and they can be overwhelming. Adjusting to such concerns as reduced physical capacity, major personal losses, thoughts of death, is difficult.

Old, ill, infirm, it is easy enough to become depressed, doubly so if also living alone. You must anticipate or guard against depression. If you are failing to do so, or if you notice failing in some other person, seek professional help. Medications or cognitive behavior therapy provide effective treatment. Certain personality traits can also become more common with aging. You are more impatient, more judgmental, more set in your ways. Friends and family tend to accommodate to your increasingly negative characteristics, even when you don't recognize them yourself.

Worse yet is a tendency for a minimal suspicious nature when younger to become more paranoid when older. It is hard to fix. Extreme examples include the belief that the person in the apartment next to yours is sending some electrical ray into your apartment. No amount of counter evidence helps, nor do psychiatric medications. After moving to a new apartment, the problem starts over again. I witnessed this unusual reaction in two different elderly patients, one a man, and one a woman, both otherwise healthy and rational, the woman repeatedly frustrating her son with this belief.

If you were receiving psychiatric treatment for psychoses or chronic anxiety problems, more likely than not, these treatments will continue as you grow older. The problems don't usually disappear or get better with aging. They may manifest differently, but you have more concerns, not fewer.

Should you find yourself unable to forget slights which occurred in the past, or you find yourself still blaming someone or some situation for the way you feel, a sort of animosity you cannot let go of, there is a three-minute treatment designed for such personality problems. Look into a mirror for exactly three minutes and consider what your role has been in the anxiety you feel. Repeat it daily as needed.

Minor to severe confusional states presenting with delirium, typically brought on by hospitalization and surgery, become increasingly common with old age. Sometimes the cause stems from abrupt withdrawal of alcohol or opiates in patients not previously known to be addicted. More usually, though, it relates to sensory deprivation. The patient, after all, has just awakened in a strange environment. It is almost always a temporary phase.

No medications are known to prevent delirium or to treat it effectively. It may take a few days, but a calm environment and the presence of familiar faces should soon enough make the confusion disappear. Returning home as soon as possible is the best treatment.

"That paradise is hidden in each person," as the Dostoevsky quote (from <u>The Brothers Karamazov</u>) at the beginning of this chapter implies, has special relevance for the elderly. The crucial word is "hidden," and the challenge is to find its hiding place. Doing so will foster contentment in place of sullenness, engagement in place of isolation, striving in place of giving up. Mental health should be a life-long pursuit.

Do not overlook the benefits to be derived from growing plants. Studies from Britain indicated that such a simple response as witnessing a green plant arise from dirt you planted with a seed is a source of joy, better than psychotherapy, better than pills. Even a pot on a windowsill can be enough, though you might prefer tending to flowers or vegetables in your own garden patch.

To Emphasize

1. Stay in contact with friends or family or your garden.
2. Discuss suspicions; don't allow them to linger.
3. Avoid or limit medications.

CHAPTER 13

SKIN

The skin can display multiple abnormalities over a lifetime, some easily recognized, many not. Rashes can be difficult to identify, which is why Dermatology became a valued specialty. In a geriatric population, however, the major problems stem from three effects of aging:

1. The many decades of exposure to sun, and to a lesser extent to wind
2. A reduction or loss of fibrous tissue under the outer skin layer, the epidermis
3. A reduced body immune response

These effects of aging produce fairly typical skin conditions, such as itches, wrinkles, bumps, and bruises.

Let's look at a common scenario. Your skin has begun to itch, mainly over parts of your arms, legs, and chest. You try not to scratch. Each day it seems to be getting worse. Some of the areas involved become minimally reddened and swollen. You think of hives. A hot shower provides temporary relief. You wonder what you should put on your skin. You wonder if you have an allergy to something. It is winter, and the air outside is cool and dry. What do you have? What should you do?

In most of medicine, history is the primary way to make a

diagnosis; in Dermatology, history is less important. The diagnosis is almost always made visually, by what can be seen. The facts that you are older and the air is cold and dry are important. You have lost sebaceous glands and some of its skin protective sebum. Your skin has become too dry, a condition known as xerosis. The dry air has made it worse. Daily skin moisturizing will tend to prevent the problem, and if itching persists, treatment with more moisturizers and a mild corticosteroid cream will slowly correct the difficulty.

Sun Damage and Tumors

Biological changes combined with environmental damage caused by sunlight explain practically all the other skin diseases you will notice, particularly so in the face, where wrinkles and pigmentary changes are hard to hide. Remember this when you want a photo of yourself taken. Have it done from above, with you lying down supine. Gravity, which had contributed to the skin sagging under your eyes, in your cheeks, and in your neck, will now cause those wrinkles to move to the back of your head, just long enough for the photo to capture what you really look like!

Keratoses (hardened areas of skin) are common, more so in sun-exposed areas than elsewhere. Most of these are seborrheic, benign, and might go away with moisturizing cream. Some are actinic, seen characteristically on foreheads or cheeks of fair-skinned individuals. These tend to be firmer and whiter, and they are premalignant. Your doctor can burn them off. Other skin lesions—basal cell cancers, squamous cell cancers, and melanomas—require a dermatology consult.

The older you are, the more likely you will have skin lesions. Some might be difficult for you to see, so look at your skin frequently or have someone else look over your entire skin area. I once saw a woman who had been living in a board and care home. After I asked her to take off her baseball cap, I saw a large squamous cell cancer. Almost impossible to miss, she must have been wearing that cap practically continuously in the home.

The reduction in fibrous and elastic tissue in the back of your hands and over your lower arms gives rise to a different common problem. Simply, a minimal bump can cause a tiny capillary to break, with blood appearing under the skin. Applying pressure, if anything, is the only needed treatment. The blood amount is minimal and will soon become absorbed, but not the tiny amount of iron contained in the blood. With many repeated episodes, enough iron can accumulate to give a brownish cast to the skin, a condition called hemosiderosis. The pooled blood has the unlovely name of senile purpura! Who wants to be senile and purple?

Basal cell and squamous cell cancers are particularly prevalent in old age, and their incidence increases with each decade. They provide an illustrative example of how cancers presumably develop. The initial harmful impact to DNA occurred in the skin from some sun damage, usually decades earlier. The body's surveillance system, the defense mechanisms, were able to correct any damage, or at least limit it. However, body defenses weaken with time, and ultimately a growth can begin in the deeper epidermis (the outer skin layer). The location is random, but this cancerous growth, once begun, will ordinarily slowly increase. When visible, don't wait to have it diagnosed. The treatment is removal.

A particularly frequent problem exists in Australia where fair-haired Englishmen, coming from a much higher latitude, settled in a country where sun exposure was particularly prevalent. Skin cancer is epidemic in Australia, and indeed anywhere where older, fair-haired people have been exposed to a lifetime of sunlight.

Skin Infections

Superficial skin infections occur in all age groups, but they heal more slowly in older age groups. Even in the absence of a secondary infection, a minor skin tear could take two to three weeks to close. Thus, keep the area clean and watch it until healed.

Shingles (herpes zoster) becomes increasingly common with age.

It is due to reactivation, usually for no apparent reason, of the virus that causes chicken pox (varicella). The virus has remained dormant in a sensory root ganglion (a nerve cluster within the spinal cord) after an earlier episode of chicken pox. Presumably, the re-emergence of the virus along a nerve leading from the sensory ganglion betokened a reduction in defense mechanisms. The location of the rash also identifies which sensory nerve ganglion harbored the virus.

Patients over sixty receive herpes zoster vaccinations to reduce the likelihood of the disease, or at least reduce its severity. It works. Otherwise, painful, disabling neuralgias are much more likely to occur.

Scalp Hair Loss

Due to genetic and hormonal influences, hair loss is almost ubiquitous in older men and fairly common in women, as well. It was always enough of a concern with younger men that hair replacement therapies abounded. Although some older men choose wigs, most become accustomed to their varying degrees of baldness. Women do, too, with or without wigs.

Although there is no successful therapy to restore hair loss in seniors, you can try to diminish loss with moisturizing creams or shampoos. You can also try to build up the subcutaneous tissue between your scalp and skull with fingertip massage. It only takes a few seconds daily, and it might promote better blood supply to the hair follicles. Any proof that this works? No, but like many things with aging, it can't hurt. And it feels good!

To Emphasize

1. Use sunscreen.
2. Limit soap use; water alone washes dirt away.
3. Moisturize dry skin by soaking in water before applying creams.

SECTION III

WHAT EXTERNAL INFLUENCES AFFECT THE ELDERLY?

The following nine chapters look at how various factors influence our elderly population, either individually or as a group. In contrast with the preceding Section II, which dealt with the essentially worldwide consequences of aging on the human body, this section confronts what everyone in an American society, the society with which I am most familiar, might experience. The fact of being older colors or alters each person's response to a variety of common circumstances, which this section explores further.

CHAPTER 14

HEALTH CARE

Although patients have many of the same ailments, problems, and complaints they've always had, the way they receive health care has undergone immense changes over the past several decades. The medications they take, the surgery they undergo, the laboratory and x-ray studies they use are now almost completely different. Patients are the ultimate beneficiaries of these changes. Indeed, they are the primary reason there is a health care system at all. Where they obtain care can be broadly separated between in-patient and out-patient sites.

Office Visit

Be able to identify a primary care provider. If you don't have one yet, find one. It will enable you to gain quick access to what has become a complex healthcare system, which, if on your own, you would have difficulty navigating.

When you visit a new healthcare provider for the first time, you will hear a sequence of questions:

What is your complaint; in other words, why did you come?

What is the history of the present concern? When did it start? How did it evolve? What makes it better? What makes it worse?

What is your past history: past health problems, hospital entries, surgeries, vaccinations?

What is your general health, for example, exercise tolerance, urinary symptoms, sexual concerns, diet, alcohol intake, tendencies towards sadness or depression?

The thoroughness of the physical examination that follows will depend upon the history obtained, as will the nature of any laboratory studies ordered. Patients with multiple complaints are different from asymptomatic individuals seeking a routine exam.

Finally, you will receive advice on ongoing health maintenance:

What should you do?

What pills, if any, should you take?

What kind of follow-up do you need?

Often enough, you are already receiving treatment for a disorder which requires periodic follow-up. But if you feel fit and have no follow-up recommendations, the ideal interval between routine examinations is unknown. Every two to four years to age 80, every one to two years thereafter is frequently advised, but there are no fixed guidelines.

A more recent development is the use of Telehealth services, enabling you to communicate with your healthcare provider from your own home. This is particularly useful if you live in a more remote location, not close to medical facilities. During the COVID-19 pandemic in 2020, such internet access also provided a way for patients quarantined at home to stay in touch with their doctors.

Medical advances over the last half century have enabled many patients to live longer with their disease or to undergo therapies not previously available. Often the patients were cured and could resume their former life trajectory. Often cure was impossible, but enough improvement occurred to lengthen months or years to a patient's life. The net result of these advances in medical care has been to enlarge the pool of older patients requiring care, much of it in an out-patient setting—-one reason why healthcare costs have continued to rise.

Routine Health-Care Expenses

As more and more medical care becomes needed, more and more expenses accrue in both office care and hospital care. The last six months of life turn out to be particularly troublesome for patients, and hugely expensive for Medicare. If the United States could eliminate the cost of medical care for the last six months of everyone's life, the funds saved would probably pay for all or most of the entire healthcare system.

Yet how to identify the last six months and how to identify when comfort care is better than medical intervention remain extremely problematic. One not uncommon scenario might be the circumstance of an older woman sustaining a hip fracture, usually surgically repaired within the hospital without complication. But when something happens, a wound infection, or a blood clot in the leg, or a patch of pneumonia, a prolongation of hospital stay results And every day longer in a hospital adds one more expense and exposes the patient to still another possible problem, a bleeding ulcer, diarrhea, or a heart attack or a stroke, each with its own therapeutic interventions and risks.

The point of the story is to illustrate how a straightforward problem everyone would treat can evolve weeks later into the need to make a decision about further care. Such decisions are always difficult, always ethically tinged, always financially involved, even when, as is usual, financial considerations had not yet entered into the discussion. And we all know or have heard of patients whose last few weeks or months of life were spent going in and out of hospitals.

Hospital-Level Care

When hospital entry is elective, it usually concerns surgery, a postoperative stay in the recovery room, perhaps physiotherapy, then home. You have already asked questions, or should have. Know what to expect, how long you will have to stay, how you will get home afterwards, what kind of home care you might need. You will appear to be on a conveyer belt, being handed from one person to another, one bed to another. It will seem to be out of your hands. But it isn't. Don't be afraid to ask questions.

You are in a hospital bed, often somewhat immobilized. Remember to move your legs, wiggle your toes, anything to keep blood flowing through your leg veins. You must try to prevent clots from forming. And remember to take a periodic deep breath. You want to aerate your entire lung.

About half the time, hospital entries begin in the emergency room where a slightly more accelerated but yet similar sequence of events will take place. The initial questions will be why you are there, what happened, who you are, and what your insurance coverage is (which may be the first question actually asked!). Thereafter, there might be blood tests and x-rays, other studies, and an examination from an emergency room doctor. Then a decision will have to be made, either home discharge or hospital entry.

Actually, most emergency room visits or similar visits to urgent care centers are for minor concerns, and the question of hospital entry never arises, but when it does, you are the same hospital patient as if you were an elective entry. You will get the same plastic bag of toiletry you pay for but don't need, and you will be given the same hospital food you probably won't like.

In Japan, decades ago, and likely in many other countries as well, the patients were dependent on their families to bring nourishments, something, of course, easier to do in a cohesive society. Whether this had any effect on patient recovery time seems to have gone unstudied.

Though impossible to do in the United States, it has tempting advantages. Look at how much nursing time and elevator space are consumed, how many people are involved in just delivering food trays and picking up afterwards, how much plastic is used. Hospitals could become more innovative. There are ways to do so. Just to reduce the large amount of uneaten food patients leave would be useful for the hospital, for the society, for the environment.

Once in the hospital from your emergency room visit, you will likely see one or several doctors. You probably won't know them. For a while, you may have trouble telling them apart. They will ask you similar questions, and they will make entries into a computer. Ultimately, the computerized entries will become lengthier and repetitive. If you ask to read them, you will have trouble finding the information you are looking for. Sometimes doctors have the same problem. (You may have already noticed this, if you have ever looked at your primary care doctor's computerized notes. It is much easier to continually enter data than to evaluate what to delete.)

Depending on what hospital you have entered, these persons in white, whom you see but can't always remember, may be hospitalists, or interns, or fellows in training, or residents, or consultants, or students. You may never see your primary care doctor. In any event, your hospital care, though perhaps redundant, should be appropriate. Make sure you understand what medications they may be giving you, and why. Understand the discharge instructions.

Most of the time, you have found yourself in a regular hospital bed on a regular floor or in an ICU. In either case, there will be a mix of patients on that unit, elderly and younger.

There have been attempts to group the elderly into a single ward because of their usually different social needs. In Elderhood, Dr. Louise Aronson (New York:Bloomsbury, 2019) wrote about her experience on a newly-opened ward, one for the acute care of the elderly (acronym ACE). It was modeled on a concept begun at the University Hospitals in Cleveland in the 1990s.

The idea makes some sense, for cancer wards and TB wards had for many years brought patients with similar problems together. But what needed defining with acutely ill elderly patients was precisely what kind of acute care was needed, and how this care differed from the same care available in other parts of the hospital. Dr. Aronson noted problems defining who was in charge and who advocated for the patient in this super-specialized corner of the hospital. She left the new ward after one week. What happened to the entire concept of acute care wards for the elderly remained unstated.

Meanwhile, discharge planners had begun working on a discharge plan from the time of patient entry. The overall goal, not only on this ward but common to hospital wards everywhere, was to find the most expensive diagnosis Medicare would cover, while reducing hospital costs as much as possible through early discharge. It's a pervasive problem which sometimes leads to patients being pushed out of hospitals too soon.

In an attempt to avoid the pitfalls of hospital care, a recent study has evaluated providing hospital-level care at home (Annals of Internal Medicine, 21 January, 2020). It clearly required a community geared to providing the needed services, but, when used, it reduced expenses, improved patient care experiences, and found no major outcome differences.

As the elderly have a particularly hard time adjusting to hospital routine, the implementation of home care is a tempting solution for many ailments, including those that require isolation. In fact, outpatient IVs with antibiotics and chemotherapy already exist and could provide a model upon which to expand. It is also a much more humane and sensible setting for end-of-life care than being in a hospital. This level of care at home may not yet be available in your community, but it might soon be.

Post-Hospital Care

Remember that your medical record not only belongs to the hospital, it also belongs to you. You can gain access any time you wish, and should you ever move, you should carry a copy with you. Simply going to another county, another state, another country, or another job, doesn't necessarily mean you will be able to retain the same healthcare coverage or that your medical records will be interchangeable, at least such is the case in the United States as of

2020. Having your healthcare fragmented, and with past information unavailable, is always a bad idea, usually resulting in a duplication of studies, more expenses, and delays in treatment.

Remember, also, that even skilled athletes need two days to recover for every one day confined to a bed. You will need three or four days, maybe more, particularly if your confinement was in a hospital. Be prepared; you will be weak at first. You may be temporarily confused. Often, rather than being discharged home, too weak to manage, you will have a brief stay in an extended care facility (ECF), where you must show you are improving in order to continue coverage under Medicare. The ECF will prepare you for discharge home, or, if that is no longer possible, arrange discharge to a long term care facility.

To Emphasize

1. Make sure you understand all advice.
2. Keep a list of all important studies.
3. Reduce hospital stays as much as possible.

CHAPTER 15

CANCER

The older you are, the more likely you will develop a cancer somewhere in your body.

Even though cancer therapies continue to improve, cancer still remains the second leading cause of death in the United States. The single most important risk factor is age, as three quarters of all cancers develop in an age group greater than 55 years. Cure, or long time remissions, are now possible with many formerly fatal illnesses, such as leukemias, lymphomas, melanomas, and some metastatic cancers.

On the other hand, lung cancers, pancreatic cancers, and most brain cancers are still almost always fatal. Curiously, the major cause of cancer deaths among all the physicians I have known has been pancreatic cancer, yet it accounts for no more than five percent of all cancer deaths. Why my experience has been so skewed is uncertain. Perhaps more up-to-date statistics would be different, or perhaps pancreatic cancer is truly becoming relatively more common as the incidence of cancers caused by smoking continues to decline.

Cancers are common, and what happens next with a diagnosis of cancer will depend upon where it is, what it is, how old you are, where you live, and often, unfortunately, what kind of healthcare coverage you have.

These decisions are basically between you and your physician, and are often straightforward and uncontroversial, for example, with superficial skin cancers. However, other cancers may offer treatment options, options which you will be unable to evaluate without professional help. The choices could range from complex, multi-stage procedures to no treatment at all. Like every other interaction with a provider, make sure you understand what the procedure is designed to do, the chances of success, the risks, and the costs.

Whether cost should matter is as much a philosophical question as an economic one. Single payer Medicare programs usually provide good coverage, but private health insurance may not, one reason why up to 25% of patients undergoing chemotherapy go bankrupt. There are no easy answers. Don't be afraid to ask for a second opinion, but make sure the second opinion is from an authoritative source. Do not depend upon the internet or magazine advertisements.

A few years ago, during the same week, I diagnosed esophageal cancer in two separate patients, one a divorced woman, the other a single man, both in their seventies. The woman told me she always wondered how she would die. Now she knew, and she wished no intervention. The man received radiation therapy followed by surgery. He lived eight months; she, four.

Esophageal cancer is admittedly hard to cure, and single anecdotes cannot dictate treatment regimens. One point of the story, though, is that informed consent is the necessary starting place for all therapeutic questions. Comfort care with a maintenance of agency and dignity is necessary for everyone at the end of life. Both of my patients were enabled to choose, and I could understand why the one chose comfort care while the other opted for a relatively slim chance of long-term remission, if not necessarily cure. All of us constantly are faced with making choices.

Screening tests for cancer, looking for blood or chromosomal abnormalities, exist, but they are not yet very precise. They might be more useful in younger patients than in the elderly, but the search is still active and continuing.

Most breast cancer screening takes place in an age group 45 to

65; the slightly more elderly, such as the ages 65 to 75, get screening based somewhat on previous examinations. If these exams had been uneventful, and the patient is of average risk, screening may not be necessary more than every three years or so, depending somewhat on what imaging method is used. Mammography does not benefit women after age 75. Nonetheless, there remains an ongoing debate about which modalities to use for breast cancer screening, how often to screen, and for how long. On the other hand, there is no controversy about the utility of self-breast exams.

One other debate in breast cancer occurs with very old women. When a lump is found in a breast, watchful waiting is one option, for the cancer can be slow growing, causing no disability, and having nothing to do with life expectancy. I actually followed women in their late 80s whose breast lumps remained unchanged over several years. They ultimately died of unrelated causes.

To Emphasize

1. Surveillance is a treatment option.
2. Therapies are continually improving.
3. A second opinion is sometimes worthwhile.

CHAPTER 16

INFECTIONS

"THE PLAGUE WILL COME AGAIN...
BEING ALIVE IS THE UNDERLYING
CONDITION...EVERYONE HAS IT INSIDE
HIMSELF BECAUSE NO ONE IN THE
WORLD, NO ONE, IS IMMUNE."

ALBERT CAMUS

Although vector-borne diseases and bacteria were known to exist, it wasn't until actually the end of the 19th century that the concept of infections being due to infectious agents began to become known. Localized epidemics, such as bubonic plague or cholera, had occurred throughout history, but there was not yet enough scientific knowledge to provide an understanding of the underlying pathogenesis, treatment, or prevention.

Even in the absence of epidemics, infections were common enough that they caused some 30% of deaths in the United States at the beginning of the 20th century. By the end of that century, deaths due to infections in the United States had dropped to around 4%.

This marked reduction was due to public health measures, such as clean drinking water, isolation of contagious disease, widespread immunization, improvements in diagnosis, and the use of antibiotics. With the burden from infectious disease relieved, people lived longer, creating the increase in aging disorders discussed in this book.

Yet infections recur from time to time in everyone, most commonly in the form of viral upper respiratory disorders. These may be particularly important to endure in school-age children, for they stimulate a healthy immune response, which guards against future infections. Indeed, the elderly usually have far fewer common colds than youngsters, although they can be just as bad or even worse when they do arise. Nonetheless, do not medicate viral upper respiratory infections. There is no anti-viral drug that works well or is even needed for uncomplicated viral disorders.

Gastrointestinal infections arise frequently, as well, often from fecal contamination of food. You've heard of outbreaks on cruise ships or after banquets. Good hygiene, proper storage of food, and washing hands before preparing food will prevent most such episodes of diarrhea and vomiting.

There are immeasurable billions of bacteria and viruses residing harmlessly in our gastrointestinal tracts, in our upper respiratory passages, or on our skin. Infections only take place when these bacteria or viruses gain access or colonize a site ordinarily foreign to them. Examples include a skin break, allowing skin bacteria to penetrate deeper, or a biliary tract traumatized by gallstones, thereby exposing the injured membranes to gastrointestinal bacteria, or when a viral upper respiratory infection enables infectious agents to descend into the lung. When such infectious agents become lodged in body parts previously sterile to them, there may not be sufficient tissue defenses to prevent their growth.

Infections can also arise when the normal balance of bacteria becomes unbalanced. A common problem among the elderly occurs when antibiotic therapy has additionally killed off enough gastrointestinal bacteria to allow overgrowth of other bacteria unaffected by the antibiotic. Clostridium difficile and Staphylococci are such bacteria, and when they overgrow in the intestinal tract, they can cause a life-threatening infection. Perhaps you've heard of fecal implants used as treatment in order to try and restore more normal bacteria into the intestines. To prevent superimposed infections from arising in the first place, however, use as few antibiotics as needed. For example, a five-day course is usually enough for pneumonia, although your doctor may have prescribed for more.

When infectious agents not part of of the normal human habitat invade, they may also cause disease. Examples include parasites and fungi, or bacteria such as those causing bubonic plague, as Camus described in La Peste (The Plague). Viruses living harmlessly in wild animals or livestock and then jumping from this animal reservoir to humans provide another example, best illustrated by the virus causing COVID-19.

The virulence to humans of any new infectious agents residing in animal hosts cannot be easily assessed until it strikes. More likely than not, however, the elderly will be the most vulnerable. They will have no natural immunity, no one has, but their total immune response and resistance to infection have also been blunted by age.

There are ways to reduce the threat of future pandemics caused by inter-animal transfer of infectious agents. These include fostering a healthy natural biodiversity unencumbered by chemical fertilizers, crammed penned-in livestock, or overcrowded human detention centers. Everything needs its own natural environment. The well-being of human life will always depend upon the health and well-being of our planet, of all its life forms, plant and animal.

To Emphasize

1. A healthy immune system provides your best protection.
2. Social distancing and masks prevent respiratory infections from spreading.
3. Hand-washing prevents gastrointestinal infections.

CHAPTER 17

PILLS

Oliver Wendell Holmes wrote in the mid-19th century that if all the drugs were thrown into the ocean, it would be all the better for mankind, and all the worse for the fish. Now there are any number of essential drugs, which when carefully selected improve the health of mankind. Yet there are still a greater number of non-essential drugs, which if exposed to ocean dumping would benefit humans. The fish would continue to suffer.

It was my habit to ask new patients to bring all their pills with them on their initial visit. Not infrequently, I heard, "I can't carry them all." Having made house calls and having looked at medicine cabinets, I was never surprised by such a response.

Prescription Drugs

If a doctor prescribes a drug, make sure the doctor knows what other pills you might be taking. Certain drug pairs are life-threatening. Ask what the pill is supposed to do, how long you should take it, what the possible side effects might be, and how much it costs. If the doctor can't answer these questions, change doctors.

Keep a list of all the pills you are taking, which you can then show every practitioner you see. Not only do some drugs interfere with each other, some could also interfere with laboratory studies being performed. Moreover, because of the way drugs are absorbed in your body, distributed, and then finally excreted, all functions reduced by aging, drug dosages are often different the older you become.

Another common problem arises from the frequent circumstance of seeing a different physician, prompting a new prescription, thereby adding one more drug for the medicine cabinet. If you have been taking six or more drugs on a regular basis, you are already taking too many. Being discharged from a hospital with a list of medicines compounds this poly-pharmacy, for often this new list contains pills you already have, or are pills with the same actions as those you have.

Non-Prescription Drugs

Over-the-counter drugs are also drugs, and you should regard them as you would any drug. Do you really need them? An occasional aspirin or other non-steroidal anti-inflammatory drug (NSAID) for pain or inflammation can reflect reasonable, common, short-term treatment. But remember, these, too, have side effects, and these, too, have a placebo effect. If you've taken the trouble to purchase and swallow a pill, you have to believe it is good for you, even if it is not, or even if it is inert.

Is there any role for vitamins, nutritional supplements, or a whole line of similar products you can find on any drug store shelf? Unless you have an unusual deficiency disease, almost never. A normal diet will contain all the nutrients you need, and your body will excrete the excess pills you just bought, yet studies show that up to 35% of older people use a vitamin, and up to 24% use a calcium supplement, money not really well spent.

Use and Misuse of Pills

Swallowing a pill can be seductive, easy to do, habitual, and it replaces the greater difficulty of body discipline, diet, and exercise.

But pay attention. The older you are, the more likely you will have a swallowing problem, most noticeably occurring in women, who have a narrower throat and esophagus. Choking happens when swallowing pills. A recent study indicated that pills exceeding 17 mm in length were particularly hazardous.

Studies have also shown that patients often do not take treatment as prescribed, mistaking one drug for another, missing drugs, or not completing the desired therapy. You might believe you can always remember when to take a pill, but you can't. Even if you've only been prescribed one medication, you will occasionally find yourself wondering if you took the pill or not. To avoid such concerns, use a pill box or keep a checklist.

A doctor might prescribe a ten-day course, and the patient takes it for five days. Then the half-full bottle goes back into the medicine cabinet, joining other half-used bottles. Usually the patient does not suffer; he or she was simply given too many pills at the beginning. But society suffers. What are we doing with all these pills? Not only do they clutter, but they invite errors, either taking the wrong pill, or somebody else's pill—a particular problem with a confused older patient in the home. One thing you can do and should do is gather together all the unusable pills you have at home and take them to your pharmacist for proper disposal. Don't throw them in the trash or into the toilet. We need to keep these pills away from other life forms.

Sir William Osler, the preeminent physician in America at the beginning of the 20th century, wrote that, "The young physician starts life with 20 drugs for each disease, and the old physician ends life with one drug for 20 diseases." He was wise enough to recognize that he was exaggerating to make a point.

Drug Companies

Pharmaceutical companies in the United States advertise their products on public media to stimulate you to ask your doctor for these expensive new drugs—-a practice not allowed in other countries. Some of these drugs duplicate drugs from other companies. It is simply a ploy for a market share, a commercial tactic that does nothing to advance public health.

Pharmaceutical manufacturers in the United States are already rich and influential. They are solely responsible for setting prices on prescription drugs, and, being privately held, they have little motivation to keep drug prices low. No wonder that drug prices are so much higher in the United States than in any other equivalent nation.

It won't change without government interference, and government won't interfere unless forced to do so. There are legislators in the pockets of the drug companies. You can vote them out. Ask legislators about drug prices. Do they support allowing Medicare to negotiate prices directly with manufacturers, thereby allowing bulk purchasing to reduce patient cost? Can United States pharmacies import more affordable drugs from other countries? Should the government set price limits on certain life-saving medications or on commonly-used medications with only one manufacturer?

Elderly patients as a group are the biggest purchasers of pills. They have a voice and they could influence policy, if they used their voice. There are groups advocating for the elderly. We should join them. Indeed, in today's world, we need to join them. If we don't yell louder, nothing will happen.

To Emphasize

1. Understand why you are taking any pill.
2. Keep a list of all pills you take.
3. New drugs are not necessarily better drugs.

CHAPTER 18

DIET

IF YOU FOLLOW A VERY RIGID, LOW
CHOLESTEROL HEART DIET, IT IS STILL
UNCLEAR THAT YOU WILL LIVE LONGER,
BUT IT WILL AT LEAST SEEM LONGER.

Calories count, even if you don't count them. Depending on body structure, age, activity level, an older person will need to ingest about 2,000 calories a day to stay in balance (3,500 calories equal one pound). It is not uncommon to retire and gain weight (more calories in than out) and also not uncommon, getting much older, to lose weight (fewer calories in, same calories out).

Fruits and Vegetables

There is no disagreement that eating an exclusively plant-based diet over your adult lifetime would be healthy for you and the environment, but very few people do this. Certainly today's elders, who were growing up two generations ago, were barely exposed to a vegetarian diet, much less a vegan one. Does it matter? It might. It is always best to eat a healthy diet at no matter what age, which today translates most readily into a Mediterranean-type diet, heavily reliant on vegetables.

You might also think that after so many years of dietary recommendations, and so many nutritional studies, we would have reached consensus about what a healthy diet is, but we really haven't. Sixty or so years ago, when elevated blood cholesterol became recognized as a major risk factor for cardiovascular disease, the #1 cause of death in the Western world, healthy heart diets began to flourish. Many came, and many went, all with uncertain benefits.

In Tony Horwitz's book, Spying on the South (New York: Penguin Press, 2019), based on his retracing Frederic Law Olmsted's itinerary in the 1850s when Olmsted reported back to the newly-published New York Times, Horwitz recounts a menu he read in 2016 in a restaurant while in the South, which he wrote, "evidently predated the American Heart Association." Breakfast special: Two eggs with biscuits and gravy, hash browns, and a medley of meats that included country ham, bacon, pork tenderloin, and house-made breakfast sausage with a "mostly grease" taste. When you look at a map of the United States concerning life expectancy, one area with the lowest is the South.

Shortly after his book was published, and while on a book tour, Horwitz died of a cardiac arrest at age 60. One such anecdote is no more authoritative than no anecdote. It is of no statistical relevance, but it is still bitterly ironic.

What are uniformly accepted healthy foods and liquids? There are many. Liquids include coffee, tea, natural fruit juice, beer, wine. No cokes, no sodas — too many additives, too much sugar, too expensive. Read the labels. Drink water, and avoid drinking from plastic bottles. I know they're hard to avoid, but chemicals from plastic containers can leach into the water with still unknown consequences. Moreover, plastic food containers clutter landfills. Please use recyclables.

Healthy foods are plant foods — fruits, vegetables, potatoes, rice, beans, nuts, legumes, seeds, whole grains, and bran. Total dietary fiber intake should be 25 to 30 grams a day from food, not supplements. A bowl of breakfast cereal, for example, can contain 7 to 8 grams of dietary fiber. And the one glass of fat-free milk added is also good for seniors.

Try to avoid packaged food contained in plastics. A disturbing study (<u>Annals of Internal Medicine</u>, 1 October 2019) revealed that every human so far studied—only eight, but nonetheless—has plastic materials within the intestinal tract, presumably from having swallowed invisible micro-particles. Will they do any harm? No one knows. We are only at the beginning of knowing what harms plastics might produce, not only for us but for the planet, as well. In fact, autopsies performed on whales washed up on the world's beaches reveal a stunning and really saddening array of plastics and other detritus in their stomachs.

Another casualty of global warming is the harmful effect on plant life, specifically the plants that provide nourishment. Barely discussed studies indicate that when plants are exposed to air richer in carbon dioxide, they synthesize more carbohydrate, diluting protein and minerals. In a sense, they produce more starch, less nourishment, throughout the entire food chain. Is this important? Are elderly patients adversely affected? No one knows; the science is in its infancy. One more reason to combat climate change. We need to insure healthy farm products as well as healthy air and healthy water.

Meat and Fish

If you pay attention to which seafoods are safe, and abundant enough to eat, they will provide excellent nourishment. Jonathan Swift once said it was a brave man who first ate an oyster, but long before Swift and long after, as well, many different fish have provided an important source of protein, a needed foodstuff for frail seniors.

With beef, the story becomes ambiguous. Most experts had indicated you should avoid red meat, but more recently other experts disagreed. (Often in medical science, once well-supported theories turn out to raise questions.) So perhaps eating red meat in moderation is not harmful to individual health, but it is still definitely harmful to environmental health. Grazing cattle produce methane gas, a large contributor to atmospheric carbon, and cutting down forests to provide more grazing space for cattle removes an important storage site for carbon. So the less beef you buy, the less demand. Every shopper can make a difference. Other meats, humanely raised poultry, pork, or lamb, for example, have no known health contraindications, nor do eggs in moderation. And the one meat you can almost always safely eat is the one you catch yourself!

Remember, as well, that food should not only be nutritious but also tasty. Being too fussy about what can be eaten and what can't may deprive you of one of life's joys, or perhaps even some essential yet-to-be discovered food element.

To Emphasize

1. A Mediterranean-style vegetable, plant-based diet is healthy.
2. Un-recyclable containers are unhealthy.
3. Enjoying the food you eat is usually more important than rigid diets.

CHAPTER 19

ADDICTIONS

Addictions often begin early in adult life, and as the name implies, they are hard to eliminate. Smoking is a good example, mentioned only to emphasize that no one should smoke anything. Drawing smoke into your throat or lungs causes inflammation and cancer.

Alcohol

About 90% of men and 75% of women in America have consumed alcohol at some time in their life. Abuse, or dependence, is a frequent problem, affecting every socioeconomic group. It virtually always begins before age 65; hence, alcoholism is rarely an aging problem. But patients who have stopped drinking early enough to live out a normal life span do become elderly. They still must prevent relapses. Alcoholics Anonymous (AA) works in an older group, also.

Some elderly, however, do drink too much, and now older, the alcohol they drink will be distributed differently in their body. Gait, speech, judgment, will be affected at a lower alcohol intake than when younger. Be careful. Alcoholism does exist.

Drinking problems are always problems, involving not only the individual, but often, more crucially, other family members and society. What constitutes alcohol abuse may vary from person to person, but more than two drinks daily every day, or not being able to go a day without a drink, is worrisome. It is a matter of definition at which point problem drinking spills into alcohol abuse and alcoholism. Since chronic alcohol abuse has ordinarily prevented most people from becoming elderly, there are no good studies of alcoholism in the elderly or how their reaction to alcohol might differ.

W. C. Fields, a mid-19th century personality, said he was going to find the woman who drove him to drink, "and give her a big kiss." In comic strips, stories, movies, plays, the amiable drunk was a common figure, the down-side never displayed. The drunk was a symbol of American culture, a foil for humor. But the reality was never humorous.

Is alcohol ever good for you? You can find suggestions that one or two glasses of red wine daily will help prevent heart problems. Perhaps other alcoholic beverages will, as well. After all, mankind has used alcohol for millennia, a Darwinian sign that alcohol is not harmful to man. In any event, averaging one drink per day, 8-10 drinks per week, has no proven disadvantages. To be perfectly clear, one drink is 12 ounces of beer, 5 ounces of wine, or 1 1/2 ounces of 40% distilled spirits or alcohol. On the other hand, there is no reason to begin drinking, either. Whether alcohol is good or bad for you is still too unsettled a question to trust dogmatic answers.

Drugs

Substance-related disorders refer to drug dependence, or drug abuse, these two categories being virtually similar, one verging into the other. Substance abuse has become a huge problem, now widely discussed as an opioid epidemic, with record numbers of accidental overdoses and deaths. Almost all of these addicted patients, however, are in an age group younger than the elderly. Yet there is an ever-increasing number of addicted patients receiving therapy to enable them to lead normal, productive lives, and as they do so, they enter an older age group. Successful therapeutic programs need to continue. Addiction is a chronic disease, just like diabetes is a chronic disease. Treatment is lifelong, now made easier in the United

States as Medicare begins to cover chronic methadone treatment for opioid addiction.

It is unusual, however, to become addicted as an older patient. Thus, there is no reason to avoid opioids for a pain problem in fear of addiction. It won't ordinarily happen, but pay attention to how many pills the doctor prescribes. You can become used to their effects.

There is also an unknown number, but presumably more than just isolated examples, of older patients dependent on a drug they may have used for many years. The drug categories are usually tranquilizers, sleep medications, or pain pills, and patients continue to receive these medications from physician prescriptions. Often there was an increasing use of the medications as patients became habituated and, in order to obtain the same effect, began taking higher doses. In any event, characteristically, physicians have usually tried to wean these patients off the pill, and, characteristically, patients resisted. It creates a dilemma, not easily resolvable.

On the one hand, if the patient is functioning normally, and leading a full life, continuing the treatment would appear to be no different from an alcoholic beverage nightly, or continuing a methadone treatment program. On the other hand, drug dependence adds one more problem for the patient, and the long term ill effects may be unclear. However, continuing mind-altering drugs as people get older is bound to get the patient into more confused states rather than better health. There are well-defined drug weaning protocols to follow, usually taking months. Physicians and patients together need to continue this treatment in order for it to be successful. Also available for referral are specialists in addiction medicine.

To Emphasize

1. Alcohol in moderation is probably neither good nor bad.
2. Drug addictions are harmful, and you may need help to stop.
3. Temporary problems causing pain require pain pills.

CHAPTER 20

SLEEP - WAKEFULNESS AND DREAMS

Most elderly sleep around eight hours, or at least they stay in bed that long. As you get older, there will be more wakeful periods. You no longer sleep as deeply as you once did. In fact, your sleeping may be so shallow just when you are falling asleep or just prior to awakening (these are the times your most vivid dreams occur) that you can interrogate your own dream. You may not know whether you are sleeping or not; your best clue will come from the content of the image you perceive. You say to your barely conscious self, "Is this person or circumstance realistic at this moment?" If the answer is "No," you are dreaming.

REM (rapid eye movement) sleep accounts for about one quarter of total sleep time, and it occurs four to five times nightly, mostly in the last several sleep hours. Dreams, even nightmares, happen during REM sleep, and they can be quite vivid. Often you will be able to recall long dream sequences, something you could not consistently have done decades earlier.

Sleeping Pills

Trouble falling asleep or returning to sleep once awakened occurs for the same reason it always did: You are thinking about personal or family problems which may have a solution, but not at that hour. Instead, think about an unresolvable problem, such as how to obtain world peace. Have a book at your bedside to continue reading in order to get your mind elsewhere. Avoid sleeping pills; they will dull your mind.

"Easy to say, but what happens if I'm already using a sleeping pill?" Good question. Many seniors have become habituated to a sleeping pill and have tried to discontinue its use without success. Resolving this, or any habituation, is never easy, but starting with the proposition that natural sleep, not medicated sleep, is what you desire, there are techniques to follow.

A very slow withdrawal from sleeping pills will be fundamental. It will depend on its dosage, the type of drug, and the length of time used. For example, benzodiazepines, a relatively commonly used drug, both for anxiety and for sleep, are particularly troublesome. One problem with their use stems from the knowledge that they induce sleep well enough, but the sleep quality is poor, a fact which also leads to increasing the dose. It is definitely a drug to be discontinued, while doing so slowly, replacing it with a different, less addictive medication. This technique of gradual withdrawal of one sleeping pill, replacing it with another, which will later on be easier to withdraw from, is the best way to stop the use of a sleeping pill or, indeed, any addicting pill.

Will gradual withdrawal always work? No. But the older you are, the more important it becomes to do so, for sleeping pills, anti-anxiety pills, and alcohol all have addictive effects, which can easily impair mentation at lower doses, and respiration at higher doses.

Sleep Problems

If you wake up with a stiff neck, it is almost always due to poor pillow placement. The best position to avoid a neck muscle strain is lying on your side, with your head on one pillow, not two. If you want to sit up higher with more pillows, make sure the pillows are positioned under your upper back as well as under your head. Otherwise, you will strain your posterior neck muscles. This partially sitting-up position is also a necessary sleep position if you have stomach acid regurgitation (heartburn), or if you have shortness of breath at night due to heart or lung disease.

Many seniors nap or siesta daily or frequently. Why not? But make sure that your resting position is comfortable and safe.

Leg cramps at night are painful, and always sleep-disturbing. They are usually due to accumulated acid metabolites in leg muscles, which your aging circulation could not move out adequately enough. To rid yourself of the cramp, you must exercise the muscle, usually by getting out of bed, walking, and stretching. If the problem frequently recurs, elevate the foot of the bed, which will improve the blood flow out of your legs and should prevent cramping.

When you elevate the foot of the bed, do not use pillows. You will invariably fall off the pillows. Instead, place a small suitcase under the mattress to maintain a fixed level of elevation. This means of elevating the foot of the bed also works to help reduce swelling in your legs from any cause.

The older you are, the more your hands and feet feel cold much of the time. You bundle up more than you ever did, particularly at bedtime. Thus, if you wake up at night perspiring, it is almost always due to using too many blankets, thereby trapping body heat under your night clothes. It is not a fever.

To Emphasize

1. Avoid sleeping pills.
2. If you need to elevate the bed, elevate the mattress.
3. Your body regulates how much sleep you need. It is smarter than you are.

CHAPTER 21

EXERCISE

The radio comic said that every time he feels like exercising, he lies down until the feeling passes. Yet, if the number of fitness centers in our cities provides any clue, exercise is apparently good for everyone. In the fifth century BCE, Plato already knew that "bodily exercise... does no harm to the body." In the twelfth century, the theologian and physician Maimonides advised exercise to "expel the harm done by most of the bad regimens that most men follow." Since then, numerous observations have amplified these basic wisdoms so that today it is impossible to find any malady for which properly applied exercise cannot benefit.

Muscle Exercises

For older individuals with defined limitations of exercise capacity, whether a result of heart failure or other conditions, what can exercise actually do? The answer will depend on the type of exercise performed and its duration. Isometric or static exercise, in which a discrete muscle group sustains a contraction for muscle building, such as in weightlifting, can actually pose short term cardiovascular risks, because cardiac output usually falls. Exercise training programs, on the other hand, which rely on isotonic or dynamic exercise, like riding a bicycle, cause a different acute cardiovascular response. Oxygen extraction by the exercising muscles goes up, and cardiac output usually rises.

How such a complex activity as exercise, repeated many times over the course of a week, month, or year can improve cardiac function—or for that matter, health in general—is not entirely clear. Although studies of this question do not uniformly agree on all the mechanisms involved, the immediate effects of exercise do become sustained with improvement in both skeletal muscle function and cardiac function. Quite simply, a more efficient exercising unit will have its energy requirements met at a lower cost.

And exercise is easy to do. You don't have to join a gym. The most common exercise in the world—walking or hiking—is free. The second most common exercise—swimming—is also often free or low cost. The goal is to use your muscles, get a little winded, raise your heart rate, and enjoy doing it enough to do it again. Two or three times a week may be enough, but there is no known accurate number.

You can find specific exercises already mentioned for your back and for your knees, but for a routine, easy-to-do, home senior workout, try these:

1. Warm Up. Hold a stretch and feel this stretch. Stand with feet apart and with your right arm behind your head. Bend to the left and hold this position for several seconds. Repeat with your left arm behind your head, bending to the right. Return to an upright position, and chin up, shoulders back, bend backwards. Then hang your arms forward towards your feet and bend forwards. Stand again and rotate your shoulders both forwards and backwards. Then, still standing, hold on to a sturdy chair. Lift one foot and pull it backward with your other hand. Repeat with your other foot. See if you can do this without holding on. Finally, stand one to two feet from a wall, palms on the wall, and try to touch the wall with your chest. Finish by lifting your

heels off the ground as high as you can and rock back onto your heels. Repeat eight times.

2. Doorway Pulls. Grasp a doorway with both hands, thumbs facing down, and lean back with your feet together or staggered. Extend your arms, leaning backwards, thrusting your pelvis backward. Then pull yourself back to an upright position, thrusting your pelvis forward. Repeat five times.

3. Push Ups. If floor push-ups become too hard, do counter push-ups. To do these, place your hands on a counter. Bring your shoulders over your hands and lower your chest towards the counter. Keep a straight line with your back. You can change your foot position to increase or decrease the difficulty. Raise your body up. Repeat five times.

4. Chair Squats. Use a chair with height low enough to challenge you. Sit with your arms across your chest. Keeping your back straight, stand up. Repeat five times.

Depending on your fitness, age, interest, and motivation, you can do two or three sets of these at least several times a week or even daily. Be innovative. Try different exercises. If a full range of motion exercise is too hard, try a partial one. It is all right to improvise. What is important is to stretch your joints and stress your muscles.

Balance Exercises

Seventy-year-olds have few balance problems; ninety-year-olds all do. One test is to get up unaided from a chair, walk ten feet away, return to the chair, and sit down. If completed within ten seconds, you don't yet have substantial difficulty with your balance. Nonetheless, you cannot walk a straight line as well as you once could, and you might have brief moments of unsteadiness. It will get worse. Why? Because balance is not only dependent on muscular strength, but also on the body's sense of position in space. In other words, if you can feel where your feet are, if you can see your surroundings, if your middle ear semicircular canals are functioning normally, and if the blood supply to your brain is normal, you will not feel dizzy or unbalanced. Yet, one or another, or all of these modalities will become impaired with advancing age.

Another way to test your balance is, while standing, raise one foot off the floor. Then close your eyes and try to maintain that position for 10 seconds or more. Repeat with the other foot. This is also an exercise you can incorporate into your daily routine. Keeping fit and balanced prevents falls and will help you avoid the need for medical attention at any age. Uneven surfaces outdoors are particularly hazardous for older individuals with balance problems. Here, too, hiking poles can be indispensable.

While patients recognize that exercise is good, older patients, however, are also reluctant to start an exercise program or do not know how to go about beginning. Community classes and television programs are inexpensive and can provide guidance. Physicians and other caregivers also have a role. A few minutes emphasizing the benefits of exercise and demonstrating the actual exercise problem can outweigh many prescriptions.

But John Dryden already recognized this fact in the 17th century, when he stated, "Better to hunt in fields for health un-bought than fee the doctor for a nauseous draught. The wise, for cure, on exercise depend."

To Emphasize

1. Stay fit. Exercise daily helps, enough to get a little winded.
2. You don't need special equipment.
3. Stretch your joints, especially before walking, climbing, or hiking.

CHAPTER 22

MONEY

Use and Misuse

There are a few, very few, but very wealthy individuals in the United States who have so much money and so many contacts or resources that they can play a major role in public policy. They may themselves be elderly, but they don't really represent the elderly. They can use their money for a public gain, they can use it for private gain, or they can use it for both.

A common example of both public and private gain derives from their funding major buildings, schools, museums, hospital wings, and the like. When government cannot or does not fund these building projects, the very wealthy can. The public benefits, but so does the donor, who receives tax breaks, whose name adorns the building, and who thereafter has access to these institutions, to their boards, and to a heightened sphere of influence in society. You and I, dear reader, have none of these advantages, even when our tax dollars help pay for their advantages.

Money in Insurance

Money has always been fundamental to your health benefits and mine. With the advent of Medicare in the 1960s, a social program the American Medical Association (AMA), fearing government control and its possible negative impact on doctors' salaries, resisted. Never mind that it helped the elderly, who for the first time could receive guaranteed healthcare. They still receive it, but it has become more expensive and fragmented. Over the years, various alternative plans have been discussed, with implementation of the Affordable Care Act during the Obama Administration the most recent.

Increasingly being discussed is " single payer," which would be a government run, low-overhead, comprehensive, and straightforward system for all elderly, indeed for every age group. The concept is embraced by a majority of doctors and patients in the United States, but by no insurance companies.

Every time the issue of single payer appears on a ballot, special interests and insurance companies, with their large sums, can mount campaigns which defeat these measures at voting time. There are always a select group of politicians who favor the insurance industry, not the best interests of patients.

Good healthcare, just like good schools, nutritious food, safe shelter, is not only in the best interest of society, it is a basic human right. It is not a commodity, and the cost of care should be a concern of the government, not of the individual.

Yet, once a year, various health plans vie with each other for patients. The elderly are not exempt, as the several senior advantage plans attest. What separates one plan from another is always unclear, but they all have areas in common: They tend to restrict choice by limiting access to providers. They cost more than straight Medicare. They are, in fact, insurance companies, and they operate for a profit.

Money in Health Care

Not only do costs affect the elderly in the area of insurance, but also they affect the elderly throughout the healthcare system, particularly with the increasing recent impact of corporate medicine. As reported in the Fall 2019 newsletter of Physicians for a National Health Program (PHNP), a new trend of venture capitalist firms purchasing physician practices is behind some of the recent increase in out-of-network bills, bills the patient must pay, not the insurance company. Moreover, in order to increase profits, the insurance companies upgrade diagnoses to those which receive a higher Medicare reimbursement. Costs to the elderly also rise proportionately.

A typical example of this kind of corporate takeover is the growth of private equity-backed dermatology management firms. These firms are rapidly buying up a growing number of dermatology practices. The overarching theme is pressure on profits—seeing more patients, doing more procedures, and hiring more physician extenders, individuals who receive little or no supervision and work in satellite clinics (as reported in PNHP Fall 2019 newsletter).

Corporate medicine is beginning to affect all parts of the healthcare system. About two-thirds of United States hospitals outsource the staffing of their emergency departments to physician management firms. In so doing, bills for physician services have risen, as have the use of such income-producing modalities as imaging studies in the emergency room and out-of-network billing. Another common example derives from ambulance transfers to and from emergency departments, the vast majority of which are not covered by your insurance carrier, and result in a very expensive out-of-network cost, billed to you.

Try to complain about any billing, and you soon discover how hard it is to find the right office or person to hear your concerns. Trying to understand your policy may not help. Private insurance plans tend to be difficult to understand, as anyone deciphering a hospital bill will soon discover.

All these excess charges, usually unanticipated, result in higher costs to seniors, sometimes much higher costs, explaining why the costs associated with healthcare account for more private bankruptcy claims in the United States than any other cause.

Money in Pharma

The OxyContin and fentanyl scandal in the early 21st century, in which pharmaceutical companies actively promoted a drug known to be addictive and which, in fact, contributed to the United States addiction problem and overdose deaths, was shocking. Equally egregious, though less discussed, are the huge profits the companies were able to make, and the huge amount of money the company owners extracted, a phenomenon seen throughout the industry.

These large salaries, bonuses, and benefits to top management have the effect of robbing lower end employees of a decent wage. The elderly are particularly vulnerable to such market manipulations, for they almost uniformly live on fixed or restricted incomes, unable to match drug price increases that larger companies can manipulate.

Big Pharma not only made money with questionable ethical behavior, but they also remain disproportionately able to influence their own incomes. As quoted in PNHP, "If Medicare had paid the average price that the UK, Japan, and Ontario, Canada, paid for prescription drugs, it would have saved $72.9 billion in 2018." That estimate comes from a new study comparing Medicare Part D drug prices to the prices in other nations.

Money in Employment

Older employees not protected enough by unions or laws sometimes find themselves released in favor of younger hires, thereby reducing company payroll and healthcare costs. Companies also switch full-time employees to part-time, or change their status by calling them private contractors rather than employees. Or companies abandon their workers entirely, sending the entire enterprise to a foreign country where costs are much lower.

The older workers, who are now newly unemployed, are less likely to find new work, not only producing an economic burden, but also creating a problem of prestige or self-worth. It is very unusual to read that top management suffers any deprivation, but their employees, set adrift without healthcare coverage or adequate income to face the trials and costs of aging, suffer. Being 65 or 70 and abruptly losing your job is jarring, particularly so if you have few outside resources.

To Emphasize

1. Aiming at a healthy citizenry is an appropriate role for government.
2. Single payer is less expensive than private insurance.
3. Profit should not interfere with medical treatment.

SECTION IV

WHAT HAPPENS TOWARDS THE END OF LIFE?

The next three chapters look at what happens as you lose your independence, as your health declines. Approaching 80 or 90 and having lost friends, you recognize that your pool of long-time acquaintances has shrunk. Some died too young. Others had already outlived the life expectancy they had at birth.

Some are now receiving chemotherapy, or are recovering from joint replacement surgery, or have a spouse with early dementia. Some no longer drive, staying mostly at home. They have become increasingly dependent on their children, or if they have no children or family, they depend on social services. They no longer entertain, or entertain much less. You find you are increasingly the one who must make the effort to stay in touch.

Some may still be quite fit. You might be, too. The future could still be up to you—until it no longer is.

CHAPTER 23

HOME CARE OR ASSISTED LIVING

As long as your mind remains alert, you are the ultimate expert about yourself. No matter your age or circumstance, you know your own likes and dislikes better than anyone. You are unique. But don't be stubborn. Listen to your family or friends. If they think you should no longer drive a car or own one, they might be right. If they believe your home has become too large or too unwieldy for you to manage alone, listen to them. Over 50% of individuals older than age 85 need some kind of help with the activities of daily living. Live long enough, and you, too, will need help. Better to anticipate and prepare now rather than being overwhelmed with a forced decision.

Living at Home

Wherever you are living, have hand rails on stairways, bathrooms, and showers. Get rid of any small rugs you could trip over. Make sure you can get in and out of your residence readily and safely. Don't get up on a stool to reach for something. Most accidents occur at home. Be careful.

Still independent and alone, or living with your spouse or your partner or a friend, you are nonetheless vulnerable. You will attract the attention of individuals who want to help you, others who want to exploit you. Be alert. Scams happen all the time. Don't believe for any reason whatsoever that it is your grandchild on the phone requesting money to be sent. Do not give your credit card number or bank account number to anyone without first checking with your financial advisor, lawyer, or bank. Requests for money are almost always scams.

Do not believe advertisements about the benefit of drugs or treatments. Do not order them on line. Do not buy them over-the-counter.

Do not automatically send a check to a charitable organization. Many function to provide employment for their officers and staff and send a low percentage of your donation to the charity. Investigate first. Charity Navigator, accessible on the internet, can be an independent source of information about how a specific charity allocates funds.

Be prepared. Your assets need protection. If you own any real estate, set up a trust. If you don't own real estate and have lesser means, at the very least:

1. Make a will.
2. Obtain a durable power of attorney for money.
3. Obtain an advanced healthcare directive.
4. Assign a designated beneficiary for any retirement funds.

Home Help

If you remain in your own residence, you may soon need help. Home care workers exist; get recommendations. Every community also has social service programs which can advise you regarding specific needs. Your town may have a citizen-organized elder self-help group. Such groups can organize help with shopping or doctor visits or provide assistance in emergencies. Join them. Use them. They frequently offer educational programs or socialization, as well. Adult protective services also exist to advise you or your family if anyone suspects elder abuse.

Women seem to provide most home care help, probably because most patients needing help are women. Men are also available to provide care, most particularly with very heavy patients or with male patients. Skilled training is not required for either. Medicare does not pay them. You must. Their important attributes are thoughtfulness, strength, common sense. Any special skills they may need are usually quickly acquired. Of course, the more practiced they are, the better. Kindness and a sense of humor help. If you find someone good, pay them a decent wage. As a rule, they are poorly paid, hence, on the lookout for more financial security and, therefore, apt to leave.

Assisted Living

When you no longer can live independently, you will face choices. Although the care of one's parents in their old age, a Confucian concept, is still honored in many families, it is much harder to implement in today's society. Family size is often smaller; thus there are fewer children. They may not live nearby. Their homes may be quite small. Therefore, when you cannot stay in your own home and cannot move in with a family member or a friend, what you do next will depend upon:

1. Where you want to be
2. Your physical and mental health
3. What kind of help you might need
4. The wishes of family or friends
5. Your finances

Catering to a wealthy clientele are fairly large-scale senior living residences, which at the high end can be very luxurious, with fitness centers, swimming pools, and wine with dinner. Less expensive residences, some with religious or cultural affiliations, provide the same basics, but no wine. Ordinarily, individuals have to be over 55 to enter these residences and still be healthy. These individuals, however, have the security of knowing that, should they become frail or ill, the residence will care for them in an acute care unit. This care is ordinarily expected to be lifelong.

Board and care homes are less expensive and are similar to moving in with a family member. They are licensed to accommodate patients, usually in small houses. They don't necessarily have licensed personnel available. Nonetheless, they are able to provide sensitive care and nourishing food. They can set out any required medications, and often they can drive residents to appointments. There may be as few as five or six patients, and the facility functions similar to a boarding house. With a good employee or owner on site, such a place can provide excellent care.

CHAPTER 24

NURSING HOMES

Basic nursing homes are there for the remainder of the elderly, those needing 24-hour supervision but not able to afford it at home. Three out of four patients don't want to end up in a nursing home, but there is often no other choice. Every community will have several to choose from, and many are good. If they have benevolent and intelligent nurses and administrators, they can be excellent.

But be wary and selective. Whoever is helping you with decisions should investigate first. Be suspect of any place that has the television on with no one watching. How much bedside care are nurses really giving? Get recommendations, and learn from Medicare whether complaints have been lodged. An excellent resource to compare nursing homes, offered by Medicare, is Nursing Home Compare (www.medicare.gov/nursinghomecompare).

Also ask about staffing. A recent study showed that staffing levels in investor-owned nursing homes were 13% lower than nonprofit nursing homes. When researchers conducted a payroll-based assessment of staffing levels, they found a still lower staffing level than facilities had reported to regulators during their annual recertification survey (Health Affairs, July 2019). It is legitimate to ask a nursing home you are considering whether it is investor-owned, what its source of funding is, and what its goals are.

In fact, in the United States, 70% of nursing homes are

investor-owned. They function for profit. Often a company purchased an existing nursing home as a real estate investment and then leased it back to the operator, increasing the rent, charging management fees, and selling needed equipment to the nursing home from one of their other companies. The nursing home, already under increasing competition from new home care entities and operating with a thin margin of profit, became compelled to cut costs, which usually meant fewer employees, lower salaries, and ultimately compromised patient care.

Nursing Home Care

Be on the lookout for nursing home neglect. There are warning signs. Bedsores, which most often develop on skin covering bony areas, such as heels, ankles, hips, and the lower butt, are often visible, as are bruises, scratches, and blisters. Failure to change sheets, undergarments, or bandages are signs of neglect, as are improper or excessive restraints, often leaving marks on arms or legs. Poor hygiene, including unwashed and matted hair, untrimmed nails, or unkempt appearance are all warning signs of neglect.

Patient care can be a challenge, from the need to monitor a strong ambulatory but totally confused man, to looking after a frail, bedridden woman, unable to feed herself. Those unable to move themselves in bed must have their body position changed every two hours to avoid pressure ulcers, not only for the patient's sake, but also because one criterion inspectors use to judge patient care is the presence or absence of pressure ulcers.

Nursing homes are routinely evaluated for the care they give. Nurses documenting and rounding on all the patients to give out prescribed pills, sometimes up to four times a day, uses up much or most of their time, actually preventing good bedside care. Nurses are often reluctant to question a doctor's order, but in a nursing home setting, the need for many medications can be questioned. After all, what is the goal? One survey I conducted several years ago indicated that the median number given to each patient was six different pills daily, most of them unnecessary.

The ideal government inspection would be unannounced visits, looking at both patients and charts with the nurses in attendance. The medical record need reflect no more than the major health problems or diagnoses, the purpose of any intervention, and any accidents or important disruptions. What percent of each meal eaten, for example, is meaningless. Yet it is often recorded three times a day, every day. Health records soon become so lengthy that their main value resides with trial lawyers looking for flaws, should some question or complaint have arisen.

A record cluttered with check marks and information over each 8-hour shift soon becomes useless. Nursing home administrators and government inspectors need to work together to obtain a workable and useful protocol. Nursing home employees spending less time recording information would find more time for social interaction with patients, organizing stretch and exercise routines, attending to the very real challenges of turning bedridden patients frequently, and checking for incontinence.

Patients who are incontinent need special attention to avoid bed wetting. One technique would be to arrange a urination schedule every two hours, and if successful, increase it by adding fifteen or thirty minutes weekly. However, this is clearly a time-consuming activity, and a nursing home can have several to many incontinent patients, all the more reason to ensure that nurses are available for the needs of patients, not the filling out of charts.

COVID-19 and Nursing Homes

Another nursing home problem arose with the Coronavirus epidemic. Many nursing homes are compact, enabling, often even fostering, close contact among patients or between patients and staff. It is meant to be congenial, not dangerous. If pitfalls to close contact were known, they were not discussed. There was no reason to expect problems until the unprecedented 2020 COVID-19 pandemic erupted.

The resulting death toll was high, perhaps higher than for any other group in the United States. There were three main reasons:

1. Nursing home patients are generally old, frail, and in poor health—exactly the type of patient most vulnerable to a new virus against which no one had native immunity.

2. There was close contact between patients, staff, and other individuals, including visitors from almost anywhere in the world. Some patient rooms might hold two to four patients, and some staff members might themselves come from communities where many family groups live close together. Such close contact from many different possible sources, with minimal distancing, enhances the spread of an infection, which is exactly what happened with the highly contagious, largely airborne, SARS-CoV-2 virus. It spread quickly and widely.

3. Nursing homes were not prepared to isolate patients with such typical common respiratory symptoms as a slight cough or low-grade fever. Could they even be expected to recognize the threat? It is unlikely that any of them had an efficient way to manage isolation, or even simply to provide masks.

Now that nursing homes are aware of the need to protect patients and staff should another contagious infection arise, ask what provisions a particular nursing home or assisted living residence has in place, if you are considering admission there.

Unresponsive Patients

Many patients spend months to years in a nursing home. Initially they may only have required partial care, but in the passage of time, all care needs rise. Patients who become unaware of their surroundings and can no longer interact with visitors or family pose problems needing resolution. What should be done when these patients are no longer able to consent to their care?

Just as in an acute care hospital, where patients might be deemed "brain dead," ethical questions arise in nursing homes about ending life support systems. These patients, unresponsive, bedridden, but still with heart pumping and breathing, present difficulties. They would have already died without intervention, and it is unlikely that they would wish to be in this setting at that moment. Feeding tubes, intravenous fluid therapy, and medications are all inappropriate. A graceful death in sensitive surroundings is equally important for patients and for survivors, and also for staff. Nursing homes rarely provide private space for leave-taking. They could and they should. Ask about it.

CHAPTER 25

DEATH AND DYING

AN OLDER PATIENT WITH A LONG-STANDING CANCER HAD FELT WELL UNTIL RECENTLY, WHEN RAPIDLY PROGRESSING SYMPTOMS SPURRED AN URGENT VISIT TO THE PATIENT'S PRIMARY CARE CLINIC. UNFORTUNATELY, FAR ADVANCED METASTATIC DISEASE WAS DIAGNOSED. REFERRAL WAS MADE TO AN ONCOLOGIST, WHERE, AFTER A THOROUGH EXAMINATION, THE PATIENT LEARNED THAT THE "THE PROBLEM IS SERIOUS BUT NOT NECESSARILY HOPELESS." STUNNED, THE PATIENT SOUGHT A SECOND OPINION AND HEARD THAT "THE PROBLEM IS HOPELESS BUT NOT NECESSARILY SERIOUS."

Are terminal disorders serious but not hopeless or hopeless but not serious? You might feel healthy, but you are old. Humor helps. Death awaits. You scan obituaries. People younger than you are gone. You have lost family, friends. You may be next. You should do something—prepare a will. But you don't. One third to one half of all people don't. But then you learn you have a potentially fatal disease. Your reactions, that of doctors, of friends, of family, will depend upon your social, your economic, your cultural, your religious background.

Trying to Understand Death

What is the meaning of death? You might have a spiritual answer, a cultural answer, a philosophical one, or no answer at all. "It is nothing to be frightened of," Julian Barnes wrote in his intelligent book of the same title (New York: Vintage Books, 2009.) Therein contains the story of Sibelius and friends, meeting regularly for lunch in Helsinki to discuss death. No other topic was allowed. No music. Nothing but one's thoughts of death. Death is serious, they knew, not to be ignored, not to be hidden by taboos. Everyone should confront this, their common fate. They didn't reach any conclusions. They didn't try to. One century ago, people were also more accustomed to death. Infant, maternal, and tuberculosis mortalities were high enough that every family was affected.

Now, though, in westernized countries, mortality rates from tuberculosis, from infant or maternal deaths, are low. When a young person dies from a gunshot wound or in a vehicular accident, it is an unexpected, terrible tragedy, not an expectation. The only death we understand is that of an old person.

Deaths that occur in far-off countries beset by civil wars, or deaths among migrant groups trying to escape their own countries, don't really affect most of us, even when we sympathize with their plight. We feel we are powerless to help. They are too remote. Their deaths become a statistic.

It is different when death begins to concern ourselves. Early on, we feel we are young and twenty and will live forever. Once older, we begin to think more often of death, increasingly so as the years advance. It is largely a private concern. We tend not to talk about death with our spouses or with our family. We should more often. We resist.

Who really wants to focus on all of death's implications? The finality is jarring. When we begin to analyze why so jarring, we recognize we will be cut off permanently from the lives of those dear to us. Permanently, a word so precise and final. The curiosity we might have about all kinds of future exploits will not be satisfied. If we are very old, we might only want to know who will win the next election. Less old, we might wonder what global warming will bring to this planet. We would like to know what will become of our nieces, nephews, grandchildren. When asked as a theoretical construct, would we prefer meeting and talking with great-great-grandparents or meeting and talking with great-great-grandchildren? The choice is invariably to meet and talk with great-great-grandchildren. We want to know about the future, a future that our death will have interrupted.

"Do not go gently into that good night.

Rage, rage against the dying of the light,"
as Dylan Thomas wrote. This poet presumably knew that rage alone was not enough. At least, it did not save him. He kept on drinking. But rage is an understandable reaction when death is near and certain, but comes too soon.

Death, however, can also be near and certain but does not come too soon. A friend, an 89-year-old widow, living alone in her own home, with family nearby, still very alert and responsible, but increasingly uncomfortable with chronic back pain, recently hugely complicated by metastatic breast cancer, shortness of breath, and weakness, could no longer tolerate a lack of control over her own life. One morning in her own home, she had a medically assisted suicide, legal in the state where she lived. She had always been organized, in charge, even compulsively so, and had already arranged for the disposal of all her belongings.

You might think that this was now the end of her life, but she had prepared for more. She planned so carefully that she had also arranged for her own memorial service, with a prepared guest list, menu, and program to be held in a friend's home four months afterwards. Only then did she really die.

More important to her, though, was not death, but that she was able to curtail dying. Life no longer had meaning for her; it only provided suffering. Her choice was her own, one she was free to make.

When asked to contemplate death and dying, invariably individuals want to avoid dying, at least an undignified, discomforting dying, one in which they will lose their humanity. Death, on the other hand, is human; it is indeed nothing to be feared. Dying, on the other hand, can be.

"The only really ugly thing on earth," Nelson Algren once wrote, "is the death that comes before true death." There are clearly other ugly things to find in life, but not remaining involved at its end, not enjoying life when you can, is one. You still have time to make sense of your own life.

Yet, when the underlying disease impairs physical mobility but leaves the mind intact, for example, ALS (amyotrophic lateral sclerosis) or MS (multiple sclerosis), patients with these diseases can show grandeur, spirit, intelligence, while trying to maintain their connections as long as possible. Their shortened life is tragic, perhaps, but never ugly.

Similarly, when patients have severely compromised brain function due to traumatic accidents or strokes, they are alive, but often helpless. Their life is impaired. It can be tragic but never ugly.

Certifying Death

Death most often comes in two ways. It can be sudden and unexpected, in which case we console the survivors that at least there was no suffering. Or it can be the end result of a short-term or long-term illness, in which case we can console the survivors that it enabled an orderly leave-taking. However, from an administrative point of view, death has not become official until a death has been pronounced and a death certificate signed.

Recently, a nurse woke the intern on duty to come pronounce a patient dead. Fresh out of medical school, it was his first night in the hospital, and he had never heard of such a request. It was 2 a.m. He put on a white coat over his scrubs. The hospital hallways were long, quiet, eerily empty. He finally found the right ward and walked into the patient's small room, where there were several people standing around the bed. They were strangers. He was a stranger in a white coat. They parted to allow him to reach the bedside, where lay an old man, supine, eyes closed, not breathing, apparently the patriarch of the family gathered around. The doctor took out his stethoscope, bent over the patient, and placed the stethoscope on the man's immobile chest. The room was still. He heard only the shallow breathing of the people around him. Everyone seemed to be holding their breath. He straightened up. All eyes were on him. He squared his shoulders, and with a loud, stentorian voice intoned, "I now pronounce you dead."

This may not have happened exactly that way, but the fact remains that doctors, just as they certify birth, have to certify death. Although everyone would rather die at home, some 40% of deaths occur in a hospital, extended care facility, or nursing home, usually in a cramped space with medical equipment, tables, and trays blocking the bed, and often enough, IV fluids still hanging on a pole next to the bed.

Nothing could be less congenial, but it need not be so. When family or friends are involved, leave-taking in a hospital should have an embracing setting, which the facility, unfortunately, rarely provides. What a difference it would make if hospital staff were available to answer questions; to help with death certificates, funeral arrangements, and documents; and to remove personal belongings. They could lighten the burden that this death had just created.

When the cause of death is unknown, or when the death took place without doctors in attendance, coroners become involved.

Someone has to sign the death certificate. A recent insert in the New Yorker magazine noted from a Victoria, British Columbia, newspaper, "I often say that as a coroner, you are dealing with people at the worst time in their lives," which the magazine placed in their department of understatements.

The worst time, of course, no longer belongs to the coroner's patient; it belongs to the survivors. Someone will have to make funeral arrangements. Someone will have to clean out the patient's living quarters, pay the bills, notify friends and family. It can be a relatively straightforward task if the patient had planned ahead. But unplanned, with a fairly large estate, with poorly arranged documents, with an apartment jammed with personal belongings or in a home lived in for decades, it can create months of work for the next of kin to complete. Even death can use preparation.

When death within six months is anticipated, hospice care, covered by Medicare, can be invaluable. Compassionate end-of-life care at home is everyone's ideal. By definition, it is rewarding and intelligent. A hospice program can help patients take stock of their own lives, and it will also help patients make choices about life's final stages.

Compassionate end-of-life care can take place in a hospital setting as well. One study of a program involving four hospitals concerned patients in ICUs who had reached a situation where further care was deemed futile. Moving the patients to a different part of the hospital allowed family and caregivers to solicit and fulfill wishes that celebrated the legacy and life of the dying patient. It relieved stress and was graceful to all involved, including ICU personnel, who often have high levels of burnout and moral distress from caring for dying patients.

Three of the four hospitals involved were in Canada, and therefore under single payer financial considerations. The study was published in the Annals of Internal Medicine on January 7, 2020, and it should provide a useful model for any institution frustrated with the terminal care of so many elderly patients.

CLOSING THOUGHTS

We get old too soon and smart too late, as the saying goes. It is a journey we all take. It begins with innocence, wonder, study, work, and ends with contemplation, quiet, peace. Everyone's journey is different, from birth to death a continuum, during which we can reflect upon the astonishing fact that there is life at all. We live life going forwards, but only begin to understand it looking backwards, absolutely every human being seeing something different.

Societies adhering somewhat to biological presentations designate various periods: infancy, childhood, adulthood, and elderly, with elderly arbitrarily beginning at age 65 when Social Security begins. But aging began long before age 65, and aging progressively continues to the very end.

We really cannot understand aging and death any better than we understand life and birth. We know only the mechanics, not the meaning. We know how biological, environmental, and social changes influence aging, and how adjustments to these changes can improve health and longevity. But we are not entirely in charge. We must always depend on others, and we are also at the mercy of climate change, unforeseeable epidemics, environmental degradations, wars, most of them due to human failings.

Improvements in public health and medical care have increased life expectancy in many parts of the world. Now in the United States a 70-year-old woman has a median life expectancy of 16 more years, a 70-year-old man nine more years. (The bad habits of men from

125

their younger years cannot be escaped.) An 80-year-old woman has a life expectancy of nine more years, and an 80-year-old man of seven more years. All 90-year-olds have a life expectancy of four more years, and even a 100-year-old person has a life expectancy of two more years.

Advancing years above 100 become increasingly rare, usually a matter of adding years to life, rather than life to years. The longest-lived individual, at least one fairly well authenticated, was a French woman, Jeanne Calment, who died in 1997 at age 122.

Not surprisingly, 80% of centenarians are women, but of all those reaching 110, 95% are women. If these figures are correct, it implies that women might actually have an intrinsic survival advantage. One theory explains that women, who have two X chromosomes to man's one, can use the genes of their second X chromosome, if their operative X becomes defective. Men have no such replacement possibility.

Reaching an advanced age becomes such an outlier that it invariably calls forth attention, if not respect. Just getting older is even a source of pride. What other age group except for the elderly will, when asked their age, tell you how old they will be with their next birthday?

Popular culture has also increasingly embraced the reality of an aging population, even as a source of humor. Wry observations or comical replies appear regularly on birthday cards to seniors. Cartoonists, as well, depict aging foibles. A New Yorker cartoon on October 7, 2019, showed two men at a cocktail party, one asking the other, "So what inspired you to study engineering, get married, find a job, move to the suburbs, have a couple of kids, and grow old?"

You can be old a long time. Yet often the changes are gradual enough that you may not feel old at first. However, by age 80, and still healthy, it will have become apparent. You cannot perform your former physical activities as well, and your recovery time from these physical exertions has become prolonged.

Whereas at one time you enjoyed America's #1 hobby or leisure time activity, gardening, and felt refreshed afterwards, now not only do you begin to fatigue more readily, you also need more time to have your energy restored. It becomes even more apparent after heavy exertion, as if your body reserves have an absolute basic requirement to become replenished, a concept that is difficult to define physiologically.

America's second most popular hobby, genealogy research, is not physically taxing, but even with this, the amount of time you can comfortably perform mental activity shrinks with age. How exactly mental exertion will tire you is also physiologically unclear. The prolonged recovery time that follows mental exertion also follows illness. After a respiratory tract infection or general anesthesia, it can take an 80- or 90-year-old many weeks to regain former health. Everything slows with aging, even recovery.

All species, all life forms, live for a narrowly restricted period of time, then die. This death is surely preordained, enabling the specie to continue with new growth upon the decay of the old, sometimes viewed as a religious concept, but also genetically determined. How is unknown, but man's life span within a narrow range of years is fixed. Make the most of it; you only have one chance.

Not satisfied with the idea that life has a natural end, there are individuals proposing life extension, using start-up, Silicon Valley-like companies. As reported in Chip Walter's book, Immortality, Inc., techniques considered or studied include using genome information or merging nanotechnology with artificial intelligence to form substrate elements. These are to alter deficiencies in blood or organs, thereby correcting aging, which in the definition given in the book is classified as "a disease." Aging as "a disease," of course, completely misses the naturalness of this necessary passage between birth and death, a passage to celebrate, not to lament. You know what happens when you stop aging. At that moment you are frozen in time.

Being frozen in time, though, has not only a spiritual meaning, but more recently a literal or physical one, as well. Embodied in the very real practice of freezing the newly dead lies the hope that future scientific advancements will enable a reanimation of either the brain or the whole body. Cryonics is the name for this enterprise, and it is available in both Russia and the United States. Bringing aging to a standstill with the hope of a future rebirth for an unclear purpose can only be viewed as visionary or crackpot. It just takes money.

Family history illustrates the impact of genes. There are families with long survivors. One measure you can apply is to add the age at death of your parents and grandparents. If the total is 510 or more, longevity, while not assured, is favored. Even one outlier in your family, say someone 95 or older, may mean you have some of those genes. You never know, for the gene remains unidentified.

You cannot get very old without luck, as well, not only where you were born, but where you were when the earthquake happened, when the explosion occurred, when the bombs dropped, when the shootings began. Can we at least limit shootings by limiting access to guns? One place to begin is in the home, where a gun is far more likely to kill or injure an inhabitant than a feared robber. This is particularly true at a home where older men or women might reside. Limiting access to a handy gun makes suicide, always a risk in the elderly, far less of a concern.

As the 21st century unfolds, endless wars and climate change are two major existential threats facing our fragile planet and its inhabitants. As individuals, our corrective impact is necessarily small. To influence change, we need a big group, which the elderly provide. Numerically large, often interested in the fate of the planet, or of their grandchildren, and voting more consistently and reliably than younger age groups, the elderly could be organized into a potent force. Thomas Mann wrote that, "The destiny of man presents its meaning in political terms." In other words, political action will determine destiny, which the elderly can and should influence.

Just as there is an ever-increasing number of people over 65, there is an ever-increasing number of books about them, almost all presenting the idea that old age is good, improvable, not to be wasted. Glorification of aging is nothing new. Recall from the 19th century the opening lines of Robert Browning's poem, "Rabbi Ben Ezra":

"Grow old along with me!

The best is yet to be,

The last of life, for which the first is made:"

You don't have to believe this optimistic, romantic sentiment, so difficult to apply in the 21st century, but Browning is comparing the binary opposites of growing old to being young.

Young people form a group all their own, somewhat like a country with its own boundaries, albeit a rather fluid one. The youth in Europe and in America resemble each other more than they resemble their own elderly. Their books, music, dance, clothing, interests, poems, political energies are understandable to each other and are largely foreign to the elderly.

However, the elderly also have their own country in the sense that senior citizens everywhere have similar concerns, common interests, common wishes for the future, and common memories of the past. They dress differently, sing different songs, and handle devices in different ways. Except within families, the elderly are practically invisible to the young. The two occupy two different universes.

Age enters even in the way death is celebrated. Years ago, when a physician friend had died unexpectedly in his mid-50s, his colleagues, his patients, his friends overflowed a large cathedral.

I noted that about half as many mourners attended services for physician friends who died in their 70s or 80s, thus much closer to their original life expectancy. Most recently, I learned of the death at age 95 of a former associate. A widower, he lived in a retirement complex, and I had been phoning or visiting him periodically. One day he did not answer my call, and I learned from the staff that he had died. There was no memorial service. In a sense, only his family knew or cared that he had died. The same could probably have been said of his birth. We are all born alone and die alone. It is up to others to notice and to inform the rest of us.

As I am writing these paragraphs in 2020, in the middle of a global pandemic due to the novel SARS-CoV-2 virus, the difference between the young and the old has become, once again, in terms of healthcare, particularly apparent. The death rate among the elderly is so much higher than among younger patients that municipalities, if overwhelmed in treating patients, have given serious consideration to denying care to those over 80. When faced with a choice of who receives medical attention, it is understandable to privilege younger patients. They have a better chance of cure, and their corresponding life expectancy is far longer.

The final and largest determinants of satisfactory aging come from the status of your mind and, to a lesser extent, the fragility of your body. There is a crucial difference between being mentally alert or not being mentally alert. With the latter, you need help, sometimes lots of help. Alert, you can function independently. Indeed, your alertness implies wisdom. Your years have gained you respect. In a world that still has much to learn about humility, you have much to teach. In a world hurtling aimlessly forward, you have much to show.

What does actually make up or constitute the present time? Faulkner famously said, "The past is never dead, it is not even past." But the world is now moving so fast, we can say, "The future is not only here, it is already behind us." What is "the present time"?

Society is disparate and complex, mankind full of all sorts of characters. You, the elderly, are a major component. You belong to society. Society needs you. You need society. Aging is part of the human condition, its triumphs, its failures, its comedies, its tragedies. You have experienced examples of all of these.

"From each of you according to your ability, to each of you according to your need," a utilitarian, moral slogan, a principle applicable to both young and old. Just as children can be viewed as young adults, seniors can be seen as old youngsters. It's not pejorative.

It's another reflection of the long journey the organism, the human body, takes, during which gradual but predictable changes occur. These changes are the aging process, which this book has attempted to clarify.

ACKNOWLEDGEMENTS

Thank you, Amy Kelly, for your excellent stenographic help and cheerful advice.

Karen Bayle, M.D., saw the need for such a book and inspired its writing.

My son, Mishka Terplan, M.D.,MPH, FACOG,DFASAM, made many useful suggestions about the manuscript.

I want to praise Lucene Thomason, my smart and good-natured medical assistant, for excellent work over many years.

But most importantly, I'm indebted, as always, to my wife Elizabeth for her superior editing, her intelligent counsel, and her constant support.

Printed in the United States
By Bookmasters

Printed in the United States
By Bookmasters